RHINITIS

Mechanisms and Management

Edited by

IAN MACKAY

Royal Society of Medicine Services Limited
1 Wimpole Street, London W1M 8AE
7 East 60th Street, New York, NY 10022

British Library Cataloguing in Publication Data
Rhinitis.
  1. Man. Nose. Rhinitis
  I. Mackay, Ian
  616.2'02

ISBN 0-905958-92-6

Supported by an educational grant from Glaxo,
and Allen & Hanburys

Phototypeset by Dobbie Typesetting Limited
Printed in Great Britain by William Clowes, Beccles, Suffolk

*(Cover: An electronmicrograph of human mast cell granules
showing characteristic crystalline structure, ×48 000. See Chapter 3.)*

PREFACE

The idea for this book was first mooted in the summer of 1988 and a meeting took place in Geneva in October of that year to discuss the scope of the book and decide what particular aspects of the disease should be considered. The results of these discussions will appear in print in March 1989—a satisfactorily swift publication which therefore contains most recent thoughts on the mechanisms and management of rhinitis.

The book begins with the anatomy and physiology of the nose and then considers the various causes and manifestations of rhinitis and particular problems such as nasal polyps, sinusitis and the loss of sense of smell. Aspects of diagnosis are considered and topical management, systemic management and surgical treatment are reviewed. Finally, it considers the problem of nasal allergy in children and allergic conditions of the nose in asthmatics.

I have been most fortunate in having such a distinguished group of contributors—it has been a joy to work with them all. I would like to take this opportunity of thanking them for their hard work and for meeting the stringent deadlines that were set in order to bring about a rapid publication.

I wish also to express my gratitude to Yvonne Rue, Publications Department of the Royal Society of Medicine for her invaluable help and forebearance, Amanda Laman, my secretary, for her help not only with my own chapters but also with the general administration of the book and, finally, Madeleine my wife who has been encouraging and tolerant of the lost weekends never to be recaptured.

Ian S. Mackay
March 1989

CONTENTS

Preface   i

Chapter
1 Introduction   *I. S. Mackay*   1

2 Anatomy, physiology and
   ultrastructure of the nose   *D. Brain*   11

3 The immunopharmacology of rhinitis   *P. Howarth*   33

4 Rhinomanometry and nasal challenge   *R. Eccles*   53

5 Olfactometry and the sense of smell *V. Moore-Gillon*   69

6 Radiology, ultrasound and endoscopy
   in the diagnosis of diseases of the *W. Draf and*
   nose and paranasal sinuses   *G. Strasding*   81

7 Seasonal rhinitis   *R. Davies*   97

8 Perennial rhinitis   *W. Franklin*   117

9 Nasal polyps   *A. B. Drake-Lee*   141

10 Sinusitis: diagnosis and treatment *V. Lund*   153

11 Topical medical management of
    allergic conditions of the nose

    Part 1: Topical medical treatment   *D. A. Wong and*
    (excluding intranasal steroids)   *J. Dolovich*   169

    Part 2: Intranasal steroids   *I. S. Mackay*   183

12 The use of systemic corticosteroids in
    the treatment of rhinitis   *P. van Cauwenberge*   199

13 Surgery in allergic and vasomotor
    rhinitis   *A. F. van Olphen*   205

14 Nasal allergy in children   *J. Warner*   215

15 Allergic conditions of the nose in
    asthmatic patients   *G. Boyd*   225

CONTRIBUTORS

G. Boyd
Consultant Physician,
Belvidere Hospital, Glasgow, UK

D. Brain
Senior Clinical Lecturer in Otolaryngology,
Birmingham University and Consultant ENT
Surgeon, Queen Elizabeth Hospital,
Birmingham, UK

P. van Cauwenberge
Department of Otorhinolaryngology,
University Hospital, Ghent, Belgium

R. Davies
Consultant Chest Physician, Department of
Respiratory Medicine, St Bartholomew's
Hospital, London, UK

J. Dolovich
Department of Pediatrics, McMaster
University, Hamilton, Ontario, Canada

W. Draf
Professor, Department for ENT Diseases and
Facial Plastic Surgery, City Hospital, Fulda,
West Germany

A. B. Drake-Lee
Consultant ENT Surgeon, Queen Elizabeth
Hospital, Birmingham, UK

R. Eccles
Senior Lecturer in Physiology, Department of
Physiology, University of Wales, College of
Cardiff, Cardiff, UK

W. Franklin
Associate Clinical Professor of Medicine,
Harvard Medical School, Boston,
Massachusetts, USA

P. Howarth
Senior Lecturer in Medicine, Southampton
General Hospital, Southampton, UK

Valerie Lund
Senior Lecturer in Rhinology, Institute of
Laryngology and Otology, London, UK

I. S. Mackay
Consultant ENT Surgeon, Brompton and
Charing Cross Hospitals, London, UK

Victoria Moore-Gillon
Consultant ENT Surgeon, St George's
Hospital, London, UK

A. F. van Olphen   Department of Otorhinolaryngology, University Hospital, Utrecht, The Netherlands

G. Strasding   Department for ENT Diseases and Facial Plastic Surgery, City Hospital, Fulda, West Germany

J. Warner   Consultant Paediatric Chest Physician, Brompton Hospital, London, UK

D. A. Wong   Department of Medicine, Faculty of Health Sciences, McMaster University, Hamilton, Ontario, Canada

Chapter 1

INTRODUCTION

I. S. Mackay

It is the aim of this book to explore the mechanisms and management of rhinitis, a common and yet sometimes surprisingly complex condition. Rhinitis is inflammation of the lining of the nose. Although allergy is a common cause of rhinitis it is by no means the only one, as inflammation may arise from a multitude of factors. The symptoms will also vary markedly from the itching, sneezing and watery rhinorrhoea associated with allergy to the dry, crusting, over-patent airway seen in atrophic rhinitis. The lining of the nose and paranasal sinuses is continuous and it would be rare for inflammation to affect one without the other, hence the inclusion of the sinuses in this and following chapters.

The aetiology of rhinitis may be classified as allergic and non-allergic, allergic being divided into seasonal and non-seasonal and non-allergic into infective and non-infective (Table 1). Infective rhinitis may be acute or chronic and the latter may be specific or non-specific. Up to this point the classification is relatively simple but the last group—non-allergic non-infective rhinitis—is the most difficult to classify further and includes such conditions as vasomotor rhinitis and factors which may cause or mimic rhinitis such as anatomical obstruction, tumours and granulomatous conditions.

ALLERGIC RHINITIS

Allergic rhinitis usually presents least trouble in diagnosis and management. In the United Kingdom seasonal allergy is most commonly associated with grass pollen in the springtime though seasonal allergies may occur to allergens prevalent in the autumn and winter.

The history is all important and a patient presenting with streaming eyes, itching and watery nose together with sneezing and nasal obstruction recurring in the spring months should not present

Table 1: Classification of rhinitis

1. ALLERGIC
   (a) **Seasonal**
   (b) **Perennial**
2. NON-ALLERGIC
   (a) **Infective**
      (i) Acute
      (ii) Chronic
         Specific
         Non-specific
            Immune deficiency
            Clearance abnormality
   (b) **Non-infective**
      (i) **Hyperreactive (vasomotor rhinitis)**
         Autonomic imbalance
         Post-infective
         Hormonal
         Drug induced
         Emotional
      (ii) **Anatomical (and mechanical)**
         Choanal atresia
         Adenoids
         Septal deformities
         Hypertrophic turbinates
         Polyps
         Foreign bodies
      (iii) **Tumours**
         Benign
         Malignant
            Primary
            Secondary
         Non-healing granulomas

too much of a diagnostic challenge. It can be more difficult to detect an allergy occurring at other times of the year but the seasonal nature of the symptoms should suggest the diagnosis, which can usually be confirmed with skin testing. Blood tests for specific IgE will usually also be positive though this is seldom necessary.

The majority of patients with these symptoms will respond quickly and well to topical steroids and systemic antihistamines and the introduction of the non-sedating H_1 antagonists over the past few years has greatly improved the management of this problem. Topical sodium cromoglycate is also useful for this condition, though it has the disadvantage that frequent application is required and compliance may therefore not be as good.

PERENNIAL RHINITIS

Perennial rhinitis is often more difficult to diagnose. The history can sometimes be helpful and some patients already have their own suspicions as to the possible allergen. The time of onset of symptoms may give a lead, for example patients who wake up in the morning with fits of sneezing, watery rhinorrhoea and nasal block may suggest a possible house dust mite allergy. Skin testing can be helpful, though many subjects who have no history of allergy can be shown to be atopic on skin prick testing and it can sometimes be difficult to know how relevant this is. Nasal challenges may be helpful, though these tests are complicated and time consuming to perform.

Perennial symptoms are more difficult to control than those of seasonal allergy. Few patients with seasonal rhinitis would have symptoms severe enough to require systemic corticosteroids; if necessary, however, a short systemic course is unlikely to cause side-effects. For the perennial sufferer, however, long-term systemic corticosteroids to control purely nasal symptoms are seldom justifiable, and are normally used only to gain initial control. Topical corticosteroids, on the other hand, can be used long-term without risk of side-effects. They may need to be combined with systemic antihistamines or, if watery rhinorrhoea is a major problem, with topical anticholinergics. If the allergen can be identified, particularly if it is a single allergen, it may be possible to avoid it though in practice this often proves very difficult. Hyposensitisation is seldom used in the United Kingdom following the report of the Committee on Safety of Medicines in the *British Medical Journal* in 1986 [1], though it remains popular in many other parts of the world.

INFECTIVE RHINITIS

Acute rhinitis

Almost everyone experiences acute rhinitis from time to time as "the common cold" and apart from "tender loving care" little or no treatment should be required. Patients may, however, seek help for their nasal congestion or may treat themselves with topical nasal decongestants. These will do no harm providing they are used short term; however, since they may cause rebound, the patient is tempted to use ever increasing amounts and long-term use could result in rhinitis medicamentosa.

Acute upper respiratory tract infections are usually due to viral agents and as such antibiotics play no useful role. Ocasionally

3

however nasal congestion may result in blockage of the sinus ostia and secondary bacterial infection resulting in acute bacterial sinusitis. Increasing oedema of the sinus mucosa leads to further obstruction leading to a negative pressure and low oxygen concentration. This, combined with a poor blood supply, may explain the relatively high frequency of anaerobic organisms found.

Most cases of acute sinusitis will resolve spontaneously in two weeks without any treatment. There is a risk, however, that acute infection may lead to chronic oedema and blockage of the sinuses and eventually a vicious circle evolves resulting in chronic sinusitis. Treatment with broad spectrum antibiotics and topical decongestants or topical antiinflammatory drugs is advisable and the patient with acute sinusitis should be carefully followed up to ensure there is complete resolution. If this does not occur, it may be necessary to carry out antral lavage or endoscopic surgery aimed at optimal assessment, followed if necessary by functional surgery to improve ventilation and drainage.

Chronic rhinitis

Chronic rhinitis may be due to infection with a specific organism such as syphilis, tuberculosis, chronic diphtheritic rhinitis, rhinoscleroma (*Klebsiella rhinoscleromatis*) leprosy, yaws (*Treponema pertenue*) or chronic glanders (*Loefflerella mallei*). Atrophic rhinitis is characterised by progressive atrophy of the mucosa and underlying bone of the turbinates with viscid mucus which dries to form crusts and emits a foul odour (ozoena). This is normally due to chronic infection, possibly with specific organisms, but it may follow over-zealous surgery to improve the nasal airway.

The nose and sinuses may also be chronically infected by fungi and yeasts: Rhinosporidiosis, the Phycomycoses, Aspergillosis, Blastomycosis, Cryptococcosis, Actinomycosis, Candidiasis, Histoplasmosis and Sporotrichosis.

Nasal myiasis is seen in hot and humid climates, particularly in India where it is known as "peenash" and is due to infestation of the nasal cavities by maggots, the larvae of a fly (genus Chrysomyia).

Non-specific chronic infection of the nose and paranasal sinuses is a very much more common condition in the United Kingdom and raises the question: what is the underlying cause? Because the nose and paranasal sinuses are in the "front line" of the respiratory tract they encounter greater attack from environmental agents, so it is not surprising that rhinosinusitis is frequently the first presentation of systemic immune deficiency.

In a series in the Brompton Hospital Nose Clinic, nine of 250 patients presenting with upper respiratory tract symptoms were found to have significant immunoglobulin deficiency. Five of these patients with severe panhypogammaglobulinaemia, who had been referred from chest physicians, gave a history of having initially presented to otolaryngologists with infective upper respiratory tract symptoms before developing irreversible lung disease [2]. Lack of IgA or certain subclasses of IgG may also be responsible for repeated upper respiratory tract infection.

Patients may be compromised by treatment with immuno-suppressant drugs or may have acquired immune deficiency syndrome (AIDS). The latter may present with a wide variety of otolaryngological complaints but rhinitis is not uncommon.

Another cause of chronic or recurrent acute infection of the nose and paranasal sinuses is a mucociliary clearance abnormality. Apart from the nasal vestibule and superior turbinate and corresponding portion of the septum, the remainder of the nose and sinuses is lined with respiratory epithelium. The 100 or more cilia lining the surface of each cell beat at approximately 12 beats a second and propel a gel layer of mucus over the more fluid underlying sol layer.

This mucociliary system comprises the first line of defence for both upper and lower respiratory tracts, trapping and removing inhaled microorganisms, allergens and noxious agents. This system will cease to operate in the presence of infection which may alter the viscosity of the mucus or prevent cilia from beating. These secondary clearance problems are common and may follow any upper respiratory tract infection. Primary abnormalities of either cilia or mucus are very much rarer.

In 1933 Kartagener described a syndrome consisting of bronchiectasis, sinusitis and situs inversus but it was not until 1976 that Afzelius [3], Pedersen and Mygind [4] revealed that this was associated with immotility or partial motility of the cilia (primary ciliary dyskinaesia). This leads to a build-up of mucus in the sinuses causing sinusitis, bronchiectasis due to failure to clear bronchial secretions, and dextrocardia (in half the patients) due to random rotation of the archenteron. These patients are also subfertile as the males' sperms lack motility and the females lack the necessary ciliary activity within the fallopian tubes.

Bronchiectasis, sinusitis and reduced fertility may also be seen in patients with normal ciliary activity but abnormally viscid mucus—

Young's syndrome [5]. Examination of the semen reveals azoospermia and exploratory scrototomy reveals normal spermatogenesis, but functional obstruction of sperm transport down the genital tract at the level of the caput epididymis where the sperm are found in viscous, lipid-rich fluid.

The nasal mucociliary clearance mechanism can be measured with a 0.5 mm particle of saccharin placed approximately 1 cm behind the anterior end of the inferior turbinate. The particle is swept backwards to the nasopharynx and the patient perceives a sweet taste. The time taken for this to occur is recorded as the nasal mucociliary clearance time in minutes. Normally this will occur in 10–20 minutes, if it is delayed beyond this it is worth taking a small brushing of the lateral aspect of the inferior turbinate, using a fibreoptic bronchoscopy cytology brush. The specimens can then be transferred to a buffered saline solution and mounted on a coverslip-slide preparation sealed with silicone grease. A photometric method is then used to measure the beat frequency. If this is not available it is still worth looking at the specimen under the ordinary light microscope at high power, when the cilia can normally be seen to be beating briskly.

In the absence of an effective mucociliary mechanism, surgery to improve drainage of the sinuses by gravity should be considered, though in practice many of these patients have surprisingly little trouble with the nose. The importance of recognising the condition, however, is to make the diagnosis and refer the patients to a chest clinic in the hope that effective management will prevent the patient developing irreversible lung damage.

NON-ALLERGIC, NON-INFECTIVE RHINITIS

Non-allergic, non-infective rhinitis is considered here under three headings: Hyperreactive, Anatomical and Tumours. The latter two are perhaps the more straightforward and will be dealt with first.

Anatomical

Anatomical and mechanical obstruction may cause nasal block and because retained secretions lead to infection, may cause inflammation and symptoms of rhinitis.

Choanal atresia, if bilateral, will result in symptoms within hours of birth, as new-born infants are obligatory nose breathers and feeding is considerably impeded. An airway is strapped into position and the baby fed via a tube to overcome the emergency situation, but corrective surgery will usually be performed within 48 hours. Unilateral atresia however may not present for some years, indeed in some rare cases not until middle or even late adult life and should always be considered as a possible diagnosis in the patient complaining of unilateral obstruction.

Adenoids may cause obstructive symptoms in early childhood and be responsible for recurring or persistent catarrh. In addition to this it may be a contributory factor responsible for recurring otitis media and serous otitis media (glue ear) and adenoidectomy should be considered. Adenoids will usually atrophy away completely by the time the patient reaches their teens and it would be extremely rare, though not unheard of, for an adult to have any visible adenoidal tissue present in the nasopharynx.

Deviation of the nasal septum will in many cases cause nasal obstruction and in some cases will even block the drainage of the sinuses by pushing on the middle turbinate and obstructing the middle meatus. Deviation of the nasal septum anteriorly may result in excessive dryness of the overlying mucosa, predisposing the patient to recurring nasal vestibulitis. In these cases the nasal septum will need to be corrected by septal surgery and in some cases a septorhinoplasty may be indicated to straighten the septum and external pyramid of the nose.

The turbinates may be enlarged as a result of the underlying pathophysiology with swollen, boggy mucous membranes, or in other instances may be due to skeletal hypertrophy of the underlying turbinate bones. The latter is particularly troublesome in the presence of a narrow nose. Surgical reduction of the turbinates will be indicated for the latter group or for the former if they do not respond to medical treatment.

The cause of nasal polyps is, in most cases, unknown. Many authors have concluded that polyps are the result of allergy, but the incidence of atopy amongst patients with polyps is no higher than in the population at large and patients with intrinsic asthma are more likely to have polyps than atopic asthmatics. The highest incidence of nasal polyps is seen in the group of patients with aspirin (analgesic) induced asthma. Polyps in children should always arouse the suspicion that the patient might have cystic fibrosis as they are extremely rare in children without this condition, indeed so rare that if cystic fibrosis is excluded, a CT scan should be requested to ensure that it is a simple nasal polyp and not some intracranial abnormality presenting as a polyp.

All children with unilateral nasal obstruction and purulent rhinorrhoea should be assumed to have a foreign body until proved otherwise.

Tumours

Tumours of the nose and paranasal sinuses are fortunately rare but perhaps for this very reason they are often missed. The symptoms of nasal block, mucoid rhinorrhoea and facial pain are only too easily confused with rhinosinusitis. X-rays of the sinuses are undertaken on all patients seen in the Nose Clinic at the Brompton Hospital as a matter of routine. Any patient with a unilateral opacity, particularly middle aged or elderly patients, should be regarded with a high index of suspicion. X-rays of the paranasal sinuses can be misleading and a CT scan or tomograms should be requested wherever any doubt exists or prior to undertaking endoscopic examination and biopsy.

Non-healing granulomas — Wegener's and lethal midline granuloma—usually present with symptoms of a persistent ''cold'', complicated by blood-stained nasal discharge. Examination of the nose reveals some hypertrophy of the nasal mucosa with granulation tissue, blood clot and crusting which can be associated with an unpleasant odour. The diagnosis will depend on taking an adequate biopsy (tiny fragments taken with a miniscule cupped biopsy forcep seldom harvests sufficient material for what the pathologists find, at the best of times, a difficult diagnosis).

Hyperreactive

Having excluded all other pathology one is left with a group of ill-defined conditions which are sometimes lumped together under the term ''vasomotor rhinitis''. This is a rather unsatisfactory name as the mechanism of all rhinitis, including allergic, is vasomotor. Here the term hyperreactive is used, though it is accepted that this is probably equally unsatisfactory for a group of somewhat unrelated factors. Despite the afore-mentioned there can be no doubt that some patients do have a nasal mucosa which will react to a minimal stimulus; a little cigarette smoke which may be regarded as slightly unpleasant by some will provoke profuse watery rhinorrhoea, sneezing and blockage in others. This is the basis of the nasal challenge tests which may use histamine, methacholine or other stimulants, in measured quantity to provoke a reaction. Increased resistance can be measured with a rhinomanometer.

Hyperreactive mucosa may result from infection and many of these patients will date their initial symptoms to a particular virus-like upper respiratory tract illness, but in most patients there is no such history.

Hormonal factors may result in the nose becoming hyperreactive. Pregnancy is not uncommonly associated with symptoms of rhinitis and the blockage of the nose with this condition can be a real problem for the patient. Hyper-reactivity in the form of excessive watery rhinorrhoea when exposed to minimal changes in temperature may occur in elderly men (old mans drip) and in the past has been shown to respond to treatment with testosterone [6]. More recently hypertrophy of the nasal mucosa has been shown to occur in patients with acromegaly.

Alpha-adrenergic blocking agents used in the treatment of hypertension, such as guanethidine and bretylium tosylate, may cause vasodilation and nasal obstruction, as may methyl dopa and reserpine which deplete sympathetic nerve endings of the catecholamine stores. Nasal stuffiness may also result from drugs used to cause peripheral vasodiliation for the treatment of migraine and peripheral vascular disease.

Finally and most conjectural of all is the possibility that stress and other emotions (sexual arousal) may cause nasal stuffiness and other symptoms of hyper-reactivity. Eccles and Lee [7] proposed that prolonged exposure to stress could result in failure of the hypothalamic control over sympathetic innervation leading to autonomic imbalance. Stimulation of the parasympathetic supply to the nose will cause it to block and increase secretions. If one accepts that stress may cause increased gastric secretions resulting in ulceration, or perhaps irritable bowel syndrome further down the gastrointestinal tract, then it would certainly not seem impossible that a similar parasympathetic over-activity in the nose could cause rhinitis.

There can be no doubt that over the past decade or so there has been an enormous increase in our understanding of the various factors underlying the mechanisms of rhinitis. We now have at our disposal highly sophisticated blood tests to investigate allergy and systemic immune deficiency, tests to investigate nasal mucociliary clearance mechanisms, rhinomanometers to measure nasal resistance, endoscopes, both rigid and flexible, to give unparalleled views of the lining of the nose and sinuses and CT and magnetic resonance scanning which can produce previously unimaginably clear pictures of the anatomy and demonstrate the extent of pathology with a precision that, until quite recently, had been thought to be impossible. Great strides have been made, but despite this the diagnosis of some cases, though fewer than before, remains a mystery and one can sympathise with the surgeon who commented that "post-nasal drip is a figment of the imagination of the patient or their general practitioner". Perhaps, in some cases, he was right!

Hand in hand with the progress made in diagnosis have been advances in management, with the introduction of topical steroids and the availability of non-sedating antihistamines which have revolutionised the treatment of rhinitis. On the surgical side the Hopkins solid rod endoscopes have aided not only the diagnosis but also the surgical management with the introduction of endoscopic sinus surgery.

This chapter is an "overview" of the mechanisms and management of rhinitis and as such is intended as an introduction to the rest of the book. It is hoped that the reader will have found that it whetted his appetite to delve further into the following chapters, each of which will deal in greater depth with their individual topics.

REFERENCES

1. CSM update: desensitising vaccines. *Br Med J* 1986; **293**: 148.
2. Mackay I, Cole P. Rhinitis, sinusitis and associated chest disease. In: Mackay IS, Bule TR, eds. *Scott-Brown's Otolaryngology, Vol. 4. Rhinology.* London: Butterworths, 1987.
3. Afzelius BA. A human syndrome caused by immotile cilia. *Science* 1976; **193**: 317–9.
4. Pedersen H, Mygind N. Absence of axonemal arms in nasal mucosal cilia in Kartagener's syndrome. *Nature* 1976; **262**: 494–5.
5. Young D. Surgical treatment of male infertility. *J Reprod Fertil* 1970; **23**: 541–2.
6. Watson-Williams E. Endocrines and the nose. *J Laryngol Otol* 1952; **66**: 29–38.
7. Eccles R, Lee RL. The influence of the hypothalamus on the sympathetic innervation of the nasal vasculature of the cat. *Acta-Otolaryngologica* 1981; **91**: 127–34.

Chapter 2

ANATOMY, PHYSIOLOGY AND ULTRASTRUCTURE OF THE NOSE

D. J. Brain

Structure and function in the nose as elsewhere, are both closely related and interdependent. They are, in fact, the two differing sides of the same coin and are best considered together. This chapter will concentrate on those points which are of clinical and practical importance.

THE ANATOMY OF THE NOSE

The nose is divided by its septum into right and left nasal cavities. Anteriorly the nasal cavities open on to the face through the nostrils or anterior nares, whilst posteriorly they communicate via the posterior nares or choanae with the nasopharynx. The roof of the nose is formed by the cribriform plate which separates it from the anterior cranial fossa, whilst the floor of the nose is formed by the hard palate separating it from the cavity of the mouth (Fig. 1).

Nasal cavities

Each nasal cavity is divided into three parts which include the nasal vestibule, the olfactory region and the respiratory region.

The nasal vestibule is the most anterior and extends from the nostril margin or external nares antero-inferiorly, to the internal nares or nasal valve, postero-superiorly. It is supported by the alar cartilage which normally maintains its patency during the negative intranasal pressure occurring during inspiration. When due to various possible structural defects it is unable to perform this task, inspiratory alar collapse will occur with resulting nasal obstruction. The nasal vestibule is lined by skin from which grow hairs and these constitute the first line of protective filtration which occurs in the nose during inspiration.

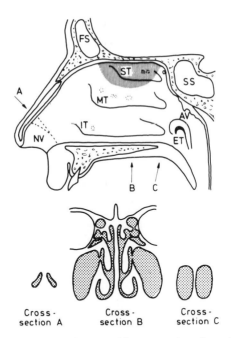

Cross-section A   Cross-section B   Cross-section C

Figure 1: Lateral wall of the nasal cavity with cross sections through (A) the internal ostium (B) the middle of the nasal cavity and (C) the choanae. Hatched area shows olfactory area. (Reproduced from 'Nasal Allergy' by Neils Mygind, by kind permission of Blackwell Scientific Publications.)

The olfactory area is confined to the upper part of the nasal cavity and includes the cribriform plate or roof, the adjacent part of the nasal septum and the superior turbinates. It is only about 10 sq cm in area, compared with the 120 sq cm area of the respiratory region. In many other species the sense of smell is of greater importance and here the olfactory area is correspondingly much larger.

The rest of the nasal cavity constitutes the respiratory region. As we have seen, this is bounded anteriorly by the internal nares or nasal valve area, which is a structure of very great importance because it is here that the nasal cavity is most narrow and therefore most vulnerable to obstruction (Fig. 2). It is a waisted constriction separating the nasal vestibule from the respiratory region and it is triangular in shape with an area of only 0.3 sq cm on each side. The medial wall is formed by the nasal septum and the outer wall by the lower border of the upper lateral cartilage. There is an angle of about 15° between the two walls and the valve area can be opened by exerting traction on the soft tissues of the cheek in an upper and

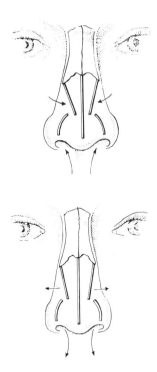

Figure 2: The internal valve (Reproduced from 'Aesthetic Rhinoplasty' by Jack Sheen. By kind permission of C. V. Mosby.)

outer direction. This is the so-called Cottle test which is useful when differentiating between obstruction due to a structural abnormality in the valve area and a more posteriorly sited lesion (Fig. 3).

The thin, narrow, irregular lumen of the nasal cavity, together with such constrictions as the internal nares, does make the delivery of topical medication to extensive areas of the nasal mucosa far from easy. As a consequence, failure of response to topical medication is more often due to this factor rather than to the basic inadequacies of the actual drug.

The nasal septum

The skeletal framework of the nasal septum consists of the quadrilateral cartilage anteriorly, the perpendicular plate of the ethmoid bone postero-superiorly and the vomer postero-inferiorly.

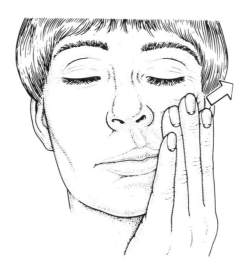

Figure 3: Cottle's test (Reproduced from Scott-Brown's 'Otolaryngology', 5th ed. By kind permission of Butterworth.)

The nasal septum is not always positioned exactly in the mid-line, but is often deviated to one, or sometimes in cases of multiple displacement, to both sides. Morrell McKenzie [1] stated that of the 2152 skulls which he examined, only 23% had a straight septum. The incidence of these anatomical variations differ greatly ethnically, and the largest numbers are found in Caucasians, with the fewest in the black races, and the mongoloids occupying an intermediate position. Many are due to direct nasal trauma, but a history of past injury is absent in the majority of cases. Here, the cause is probably due to moulding pressures which occur during pregnancy or to birth trauma, as has been postulated by Lindsay Gray [2] (Figs. 4, 5). The neonatal septum is displaced from the mid-line in these patients and the deviations are then accentuated during the subsequent growth period. In the vast majority of cases, the degree of septal deviation is not severe enough to cause any obstruction and minor degrees can, therefore, be considered to be the norm rather than the exception. Cottle has classified septal deviations as:

1. *A simple deviation*
   Here there is a mild deflection of the septum which does not cause obstruction. The majority of Caucasians have this type of septum and it certainly does not require any surgical treatment.

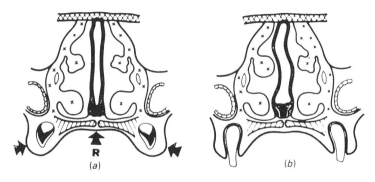

Figure 4: Combined septal deformity resulting from moulding pressures. (Reproduced from Scott-Brown's 'Otolaryngology' 5th ed. By kind permission of Butterworth.)

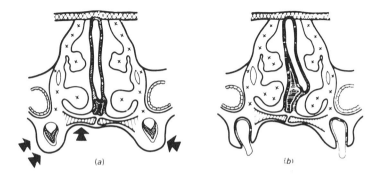

Figure 5: Septal deformity resulting from unequal moulding pressures. (Reproduced from Scott-Brown's 'Otolaryngology' 5th ed. By kind permission of Butterworth.)

2. *Obstruction*

   This is a more severe deviation of the nasal septum which may touch the lateral wall of the nose, but on vasoconstriction, however, the turbinates shrink away from the septum.

3. *Impaction*

   This is a very marked angulation of the septum with a spur which lies in contact with the lateral nasal wall, even after the application of a vasoconstrictor. This is an absolute indication for surgical treatment.

The effects of the septal deviation depend on its position, and when the lesion occurs in a very narrow part of the nasal cavity such as the internal nares or valve area, even relatively minor deviations can easily cause obstructive symptoms and require surgical straightening.

Lateral nasal wall

The lateral nasal wall of the nasal cavity is dominated by three horizontal projections which are described in the clinical literature as turbinates and in the anatomical literature as nasal conchae. The inferior turbinate is much the largest and is a separate bone, whereas the medium-sized middle turbinate and the small superior turbinate are merely medical projections from the ethmoid bones (Fig. 1). The turbinates greatly increase the surface area of the nasal cavity and this allows much greater contact between the unfiltered, unconditioned, inspired air, and the functional nasal mucosa.

Below and lateral to each of the respective turbinates are found the inferior, middle and superior nasal meati. The naso-lacrimal duct enters the nasal cavity through the inferior nasal meatus and consequent nasal disease in this area can block the duct and lead to epiphora. The frontal, maxillary and anterior ethmoidal sinuses drain into the middle nasal meatus, whereas the posterior ethmoidal sinuses drain into the superior meatus and the sphenoid sinus into the sphenoid-ethmoidal recess (Figs. 6, 7). These areas are, therefore, of critical importance to the ventilation and drainage of the nasal sinuses. The draining ostium of each sinus is usually 3–4 mm in diameter, but it has been found that an ostium size of less than 2.5 mm predisposes to infection. Allergic diseases cause mucosal oedema, which can easily narrow the ostium, and the recent development of nasal endoscopy has shown that quite small anatomical anomalies and/or pathological lesions in this area which are not visible on routine rhinoscopy, can often interfere with the drainage of the sinuses and lead to the development of sinus infection. These infections often respond inadequately to antibiotic therapy and usually require surgical treatment which is often of a very minor type to effect a complete cure. Typical anatomical anomalies of this type include the so-called paradoxical middle turbinate which has a reverse curve, and the gross widening of the middle turbinate occurring when it contains an air cell (concha bullosa). These lesions produce gross narrowing of the middle nasal meatus (Figs. 8, 9).

Most cases of sinusitis result from infection spreading from the cavity of the nose. However, in the case of the maxillary sinuses,

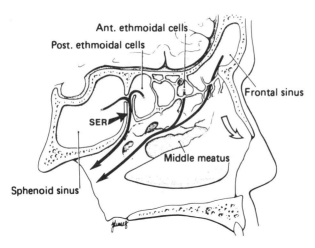

Figure 6: Diagram of lateral nasal wall demonstrating mucociliary flow. (Reproduced from 'Paranasal Sinuses; CT Imaging Requirements for Endoscopic Surgery' by Zinreich *et al*. By kind permission of 'Radiology'.)

probably up to 5% are dental in origin. The roots of the upper teeth are often in very close contact with the floor of this sinus, and as a consequence an apical dental abscess can easily be spread upwards to involve the sinus. Likewise, there is always a risk that dental extractions in this area can lead to the development of an oro-antral fistula.

Blood supply to the nose

The blood supply of the nose is very profuse and is of considerable importance when considering both normal nasal physiology and the various disease processes which occur in the nose. The two main feeding arteries are the spheno-palatine posteriorly, which is a branch of the external carotid system; and the anterior ethmoidal artery antero-superiorly, which comes via the internal carotid system through its ophthalmic branch. These arteries converge on the antero-inferior part of the septum where they anastomose with the nasal branches of both the superior labial artery and the greater palatine artery. This area is usually known on the continent of Europe as Kiesselbach's area, and in the English-speaking countries more often as Little's area; 70% of nose bleeds come from this area.

17

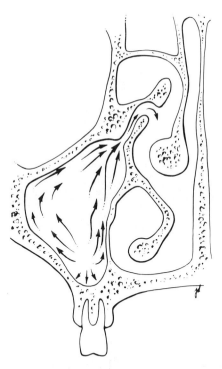

Figure 7: Mucociliary clearance from the maxillary sinus. (Reproduced from 'Paranasal Sinuses: CT Imaging Requirements for Endoscopic Surgery', by Zinreich *et al*. By kind permission of 'Radiology'.)

THE ULTRASTRUCTURE OF THE NOSE

The working tissue of the nose is its lining mucous membrane and a fairly detailed histological study of this vitally important structure is necessary before a clear understanding of nasal function and immunology can be obtained. The nasal mucosa is capable of enormous physiological and pathological variations in thickness due to its vascularity and to the looseness of its submucosa. The potential for distension and swelling is maximal on the lateral wall of the nose. It is therefore at the lateral wall of the nose that one finds the greatest evidence of mucosal disease such as allergy, infection and nasal polyposis. The more generalised oedema found in allergy and infection causes a considerable and obvious enlargement of the turbinates. Polypi are evidence of a more localised oedematous process which more commonly affects the mucosal lining of the middle and superior nasal meati.

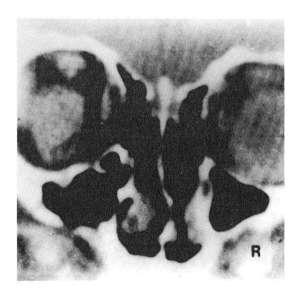

Figure 8: Tomogram showing concha bullosa (Reproduced from 'Paranasal Sinuses; CT Imaging Requirements for Endoscopic Surgery' by Zinreich *et al*. By kind permission of 'Radiology'.)

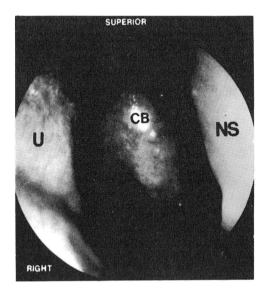

Figure 9: Endoscopic view of anterior surface of concha bullosa (Reproduced from 'Paranasal Sinuses; CT Imaging Requirements for Endoscopic Surgery' by Zinreich *et al*. By kind permission of 'Radiology'.)

19

The olfactory area is confined to the upper part of the nasal cavity, the rest of which is divided into the nasal vestibule and the respiratory region. The vestibule is lined by skin, whereas the posterior 80% of the respiratory region is lined by a columnar, ciliated mucous membrane. A transitional and sparsely ciliated columnar epithelium is found in the intermediate area. It is, however, with the ciliated columnar mucosa that we are primarily concerned.

Columnar ciliated epithelium

Superficially this consists of a pseudo-stratified columnar epithelium resting on a basement membrane which separates it from the underlying submucosa or lamina propria.

The epithelium consists of ciliated columnar cells, non-ciliated columnar cells, goblet cells and basal cells. The basal cells are the primitive cells from which the columnar and goblet cells develop. They lie on the basement mucous membrane, but do not reach the surface of the epithelium (Fig. 10).

Goblet cells constitute the glandular element of the epithelial layer. These are unicellular mucous glands with a basal nucleus. Numerous droplets of mucus are produced in the more superficial part of the cell before being expelled into the nasal cavity where a protective layer of mucus is found over the surface of the nasal mucosa. This layer of mucus is important in relation to the filtration function of the nose and its immunological protective mechanisms. Below this layer of mucus, the surface epithelial cells are all bound together by terminal bars which form another protective seal.

All the columnar cells are covered by short finger-like projections from their superficial surfaces called microvilli. Three to four hundred are found on each cell and the size is about one-third that of the average cilium. These microvilli are incapable of active movement and are not precursors of the cilia. They do, however, greatly increase the surface area of the epithelium and prevent drying of its surface. Mygind has used the analogy of the garden lawn which keeps the morning dew much better than a surfaced road.

Most, but not all, of the columnar epithelial cells are ciliated. Probably 50–100 of these vitally important structures project for 4–6 μm from the surface of each cell. They are long, thin and mobile and have a diameter of 0.33 μm. The structural framework of each

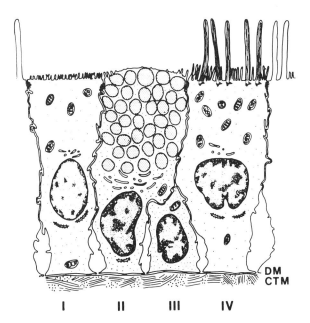

DM
CTM

I   II   III   IV

Figure 10: Transmission electron microscopic diagram of the four cell types in nasal respiratory epithelium. (Reproduced from 'Nasal Allergy' by N. Mygind, by kind permission of Blackwell Scientific Publications.)

cilium consists of a ring of nine doublet microtubules surrounding two single central microtubules (Fig. 11). The breakdown of adenosine tri-phosphate (ATP) by the enzyme dynein provides the energy for ciliary movement. Dynein arms or projections are found associated with the nine outer doublet microtubules. Rarely these dynein arms are absent, and this is found in cases of Kartagener's syndrome (sinusitis, bronchiectasis and situs inversus).

Satir [3] has postulated a sliding-microtubule hypothesis for ciliary motion in which the energy is provided by the dynein arms and this results in movement of the peripheral microtubules which slide past one another. The shear resistance in the cilium causes the sliding to be extended into a bending movement. The cilia project into the layer of mucus which has an outer viscous gel phase. The mucous blanket is propelled backwards by ciliary activity. Each beat of the cilium consists of a rapid propulsive stroke followed by a slower recovery phase (Fig. 12). The ciliary beat frequency is 10–15 beats per second and the mucus flows from the front to the back of the nose in about 5–20 minutes, as shown by the saccharin test. Mucus from each of the sinuses passes through its draining ostium

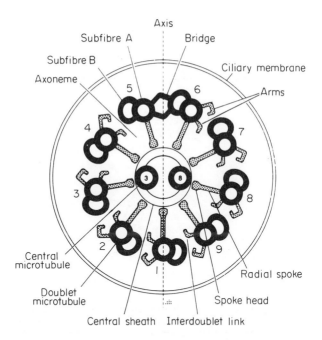

Axis
Subfibre A
Bridge
Subfibre B
Ciliary membrane
Axoneme
5
6
Arms
4
7
3
8
Central
microtubule
2
9
Radial spoke
Doublet
microtubule
1
Spoke head
Central sheath   Interdoublet link

Figure 11: Diagram of cilium cross section (Reproduced from 'Nasal Allergy' by N. Mygind, by kind permission of Blackwell Scientific Publications.)

on to the lateral wall of the nose, where it joins the main nasal mucus screen passing backwards into the nasopharynx around the orifice of the eustachian tube before being swallowed (Fig. 13).

Ciliary activity is depressed by drying and also by the damage produced by nasal infections. Messerklinger has also shown that it is absent in structural abnormalities of the nose where two opposing mucosal surfaces come into direct contact. Local applications to the mucosa can affect ciliary activity. Extremes of pH and some drugs such as adrenaline and cocaine, both of which are widely used in rhinological practice, do produce a paralysis of ciliary activity.

The submucosa

The main components of this layer include the various glands, the blood vessels and the numerous extravascular cells, which have important protective and immunological functions.

The submucosa is a fairly loose connective tissue with some collagen and very few elastic fibrils. The ground substance is a gel

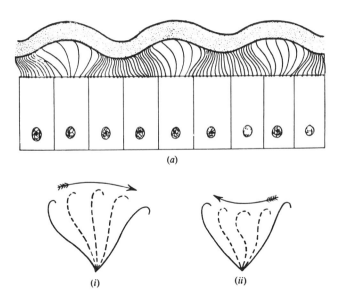

(a)

(i)   (ii)

Figure 12: (a) Diagram of ciliated cells with overlying mucous blanket. Mucous blanket consists of outer layer of viscid mucus resting on a thin layer of serous fluid (b) Diagram of ciliary action i. propulsive stroke ii. recovery stroke (Reproduced from Scott Brown's 'Diseases of the Ear, Nose and Throat' 3rd ed. By kind permission of Butterworth.)

composed mainly of mucopolysaccharides, with water, electrolytes and serum proteins forming the tissue fluids. The tissue fluid content can be abnormally high in some pathological conditions of the nasal mucosa such as polyposis. Connective tissue cells such as fibroblasts, fibrocytes and histiocytes are found in the submucosa in addition to many other cells which play an important role in the immunological mechanism of the nose such as mast cells, plasma cells, eosinophils, lymphocytes, neutrophils, leucocytes and macrophages. The full details of nasal immunology and immunopathology are given in a later chapter, but in this account of the ultrastructure of the mucosa, a brief description of the mast cells and the plasma cells will now be given.

Mast cells are found in all layers of the submucosa but are only very rarely in the epithelium or nasal secretions. They are large cells averaging 15–20 μm in diameter and have an oval centrally placed nucleus (Fig. 14). Their chief feature, however, is the presence of about 200 granules which are scattered throughout the cytoplasm. These granules stain Toluidine blue and are characterised by whorls and scrolls. They contain histamines and other powerful mediators

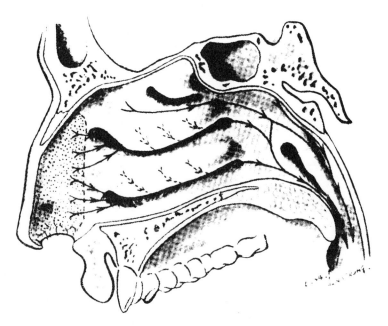

Figure 13: Pathways of clearance of mucus from lateral wall of nose. (Reproduced from Scott Brown's 'Diseases of the Ear, Nose and Throat' 3rd ed. By kind permission of Butterworth.)

of the allergic reaction. The function of these cells in the normal non-allergic individual is unknown, but they play a very important role in the immunopathology of allergy.

The plasma cells are also quite large, are egg shaped and have an eccentrically placed nucleus. The cytoplasm contains an abundance of RNA-containing ribosomes from which antibodies are synthesised.

The submucosal glands consist of the anterior serous glands and the more widespread small seromucinous glands. There are about 100–150 glands in the anterior serous group which open into the upper part of the internal nares. They appear to secrete a watery fluid with a high protein content.

The seromucinous glands are widely distributed throughout the entire respiratory region. They include distal serous tubules with more central mucous tubules which drain into a collecting, and finally a ciliated duct, before discharging their secretions into the nasal cavity. The serous solution has a high protein content and the collecting duct has the capacity to modify and control the iron and water content of the glandular secretions. The protein content of the

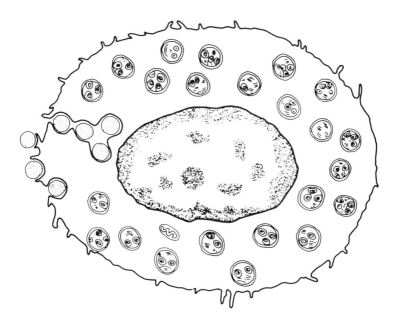

Figure 14: Mast cell with secretory granules showing laminar structure with whorls and scrolls. (Reproduced from 'Nasal Allergy' by N. Mygind by kind permission of Blackwell Scientific Publications.)

serous tubule secretions contain the bacteriolytic enzyme, lysozyme, in addition to lactoferrin, which has the capacity to remove heavy metal ions and prevent the growth of certain bacteria such as staphylococci and pseudomonas. The plasma cells around the seromucinous glands produce the immunoglobulin IgA, which is discharged into the duct system of the glands, and as a result, IgA is the principal immunoglobulin to be found in nasal secretions. A layer of protective IgA then covers the outer surface of the nasal mucosa and constitutes a first line of defence against microorganisms. IgA deficiency is usually found in atopic individuals and, according to Southill, this leads to a secondary over-activity of the IgE system. IgE is only found in extremely minute amounts in normal individuals, but its levels are very greatly raised in atopic subjects.

The main constituent of nasal fluid is, of course water (95–97%), but it also contains mucin (2.5–3%) and electrolytes (1–2%). Normal nasal secretions are clear and slightly viscous and it used to be taught that any colouration of the nasal discharge usually indicated active infection. However, a yellow colouration of the discharge can indicate a raised protein content and this is sometimes found in allergic disorders which are not complicated by secondary infection. A green colouration is due to the enzyme verdoperoxidase released from dead leucocytes which are found in active nasal infections. The secretomotor nerve supply to the nose is parasympathetic. These fibres are derived from the facial nerve and reach the nasal mucosa via the vidian nerve.

Blood vessels

The nasal mucosa is a very vascular membrane and its total blood flow per cubic centimetre of tissue is greater than in muscle, brain and liver [4]. Some degree of pathological behaviour of the blood vessels is found in all cases of rhinitis, although the term in ''vasomotor'' rhinitis is usually reserved for patients suffering from symptoms indistinguishable from allergic rhinitis, in whom no immunological evidence of an allergic cause can be found (Fig. 15).

A distinctive characteristic of the nasal blood vessels is their extreme porosity. This is produced by defects or fenestra in the lining endothelial basement membrane. This facilitates a very rapid passage of fluid through the vascular wall and also makes the absorption of drugs such as sympathomimetic agents, histamine and corticosteroids, both easy and rapid.

Blood, in addition to flowing from arteries, through the capillary network and into the venules, can also be directed straight from the arteries through the arteriovenous anastomoses into the venous system. Angaard [5] has shown in the cat that 60% of the blood flow is normally shunted through arteriovenous anastomoses.

Erectile tissue in the form of cavernous sinusoids are found between the capillaries and the venules. These potentially cavernous structures are usually in an empty contracted state. The walls of these vessels contain smooth muscle cells whose activities are usually controlled by the autonomic nervous system. These sinusoids are normally constricted by a continuous sympathetic stimulation, but they can dilate when this tone is lost and also parasympathetic stimulation produces some vascular dilatation. The concentration of sinusoids is most marked in the mucosa covering the inferior and middle turbinates and, when gorged with blood, they produce an enormous increase in the thickness of the nasal mucosa with a resulting obstruction of the airway.

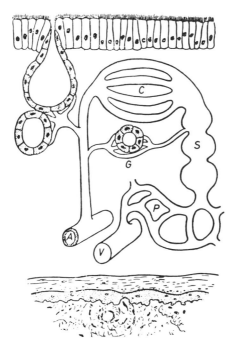

Figure 15: Simplified diagram showing arrangement of blood vessels in nasal mucosa. (Reproduced from Scott Brown's 'Diseases of the Ear, Nose and Throat' 3rd ed. By kind permission of Butterworth.)

FUNCTION OF THE NOSE

Airway

Normal breathing occurs through the nose, which has the task of filtering, warming and humidifying the inspired air, which is later delivered to the lungs in an optimal state. The nose also helps to protect the lower respiratory tract and all these valuable functions are lost when breathing occurs through the mouth. Nasal breathing is obligatory in the neonate, due to the somewhat different anatomy at this age and as a consequence bilateral choanal atresia causes an alarming and life-threatening degree of respiratory obstruction in the newborn. The respiratory and expiratory air currents are shown in the diagrams (Fig. 16).

Usually about 10% of the inspired air reaches the olfactory area of the nose during normal breathing, although this can be increased to 20% with sniffing. A selective obstruction in the upper nasal cavities

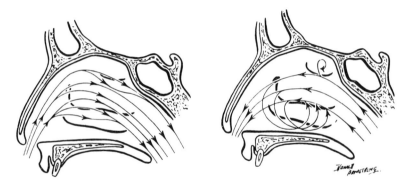

Figure 16: Diagram of inspiratory and expiratory air current. (Reproduced from Scott Brown's 'Diseases of the Ear, Nose and Throat' 3rd ed. By kind permission of Butterworth.)

could, therefore, rob the patient of his sense of smell, without obstructing the main nasal airway. Nasal breathing makes heavy commitments on the lining mucous membrane of the nose which, if excessive, can change to the squamous epithelial type. It may be for this reason that a nasal cycle can be detected in 80% of the population. Here, there is a cyclic and alternate obstruction occurring every four or twelve hours. One side of the nose will block off due to the engorgement of the erectile sinusoids in the turbinates and there will be shrinkage of the mucosa on the opposite side through which all breathing takes place. Nasal secretions are cyclic, being greatest from the unobstructed side. This cycle is controlled by the autonomic nervous system and passes unnoticed by most people. It could, however, give rise to the phenomenon of "paradoxical nasal obstruction". This was described by Arbour and Kern [6] in which these patients have a longstanding, fixed, unilateral nasal obstruction, to which they have become accustomed and of which they are no longer aware. The mucosal swelling associated with the nasal cycle does result in an additional intermittent nasal obstruction on the normal side of the nose, and this becomes the dominant symptom to be appreciated by the patient.

Heating and humidification

The glandular and vascular elements of the nose evidently warm and humidify the inspired air. When the air reaches the nasopharynx it is normally 31°C and 95% saturated. This performance is maintained despite gross changes in environmental conditions.

Filtration

The alveoli are extremely delicate and may be damaged by particles in the inspired air. An important function of the nose is to filter off these contaminants. The shape of the nasal cavities favour this process because they ensure the maximum contact between line mucosa and inspired air with a slit-like lumen, with a major constriction at the internal nares. This produces turbulence with deposition of particles on the mucus blanket which covers the nasal mucosa. Here the particles adhere to the viscid mucus, which is transported like a conveyor belt by ciliary action in a backwards direction into the nasopharynx and is then swallowed. In addition to this mechanical process there are also protective immunological mechanisms.

The nose is extremely effective in filtering off particles down to a size of μm. Particles below this size pass through the nose and into the lungs and this has an important bearing on whether an atopic patient develops asthma or allergic rhinitis. Sensitivity to smaller allergens, such as fungal spores (3–5 μm) usually causes an asthmatic condition, whereas the larger allergens, such as grass pollens (30μm) are filtered off in the nose and this results in the development of an allergic rhinitis.

Sense of smell

This subject will be covered in detail in Chapter 5.

The nose and voice

Phonation arises in the larynx but the primary laryngeal sounds are modified by the resonance which occurs in the nose, pharynx, oral cavity and lips. The nasal cavities are closed off by the soft palate during the production of most sounds, but nasal resonance is necessary for such consonants as 'm' and 'n'. A reduction of nasal resonance occurs when the nose is obstructed and this results in rhinolalia clausa. Excessive nasal resonance causes rhinolalia aperta, which occurs when there are defects in the nasopharyngeal sphincter, such as are present in cases of cleft palate.

Nasal reflexes

The nose is both the afferent and efferent component of several reflexes which are often of clinical importance, because many patients with nasal symptoms often have an abnormally labile mucosa which reacts in an exaggerated fashion to these stimuli. The main reflexes in the nose are:

1. Intense chemical, thermal or physical stimulation of the nose produces sneezing and in extreme cases this can progress to closure of the laryngeal sphincter with intense vasoconstriction of skin, muscles and viscera.
2. Exertion causes intense vasoconstriction of the nasal mucosa, and it is for this reason that exercise is used prior to making nasal resistance tests on the nose in order to differentiate between blockage due to structural defects and those due to mucosal swelling.
3. Heating the general skin surface causes nasal vasodilation and this, together with the dryness of the air, can lead to nasal symptoms which are often found in those who are working in such environments as a hot, air-conditioned office without humidification.
4. Cooling of the general skin surface produces a vasoconstriction with clearing of the nasal passage.
5. Increasing the airflow through one side of the nose results in increased ventilation of the homolateral lung.
6. Burrows and Eccles [7] have shown that when an individual lies on his side this produces vasodilation in the lower nasal cavity with often a sensation of blockage and vasoconstriction in the upper nasal cavity.

Endocrine and psychological factors

Some hormones have quite dramatic effects on the nasal mucosa. The action may be more on disease states, such as is accomplished by the corticosteroids which have a dramatic effect on the inflammatory process which is present in many types of rhinitis. In other examples, the effects are on the normal mucosa. Hypothyroidism may cause nasal obstruction due to the deposition of mucopolysaccharides in the extracellular spaces of the submucosa. The sex hormones can have profound effects on the nasal mucosa. Oestrogens produce nasal congestion and for this reason have been used in the treatment of atrophic rhinitis. Certainly, changes in the mucosa can occur during menstruation and pregnancy. Some of the higher dose oestrogen contraceptives can produce an iatrogenic rhinitis. Also, the syndrome of "honeymoon" rhinitis has been described by Watson Williams [8], where severe nasal symptoms occur during moments of sexual excitement. The nasal mucosa also reacts to certain psychological states. Anger produces a sympathomimetic reaction with vasoconstriction and reduced secretory activity, whereas such emotions as resentment and possibly depression, have the opposite effect, inducing obstruction with excessive nasal discharge and sneezing.

Nasal sinuses

The function of the nasal sinuses is unknown.

REFERENCES

1. McKenzie M. *Manual of diseases of the nose and throat*. London: Churchill, 1880; 432.
2. Gray LP. Early treatment of septal deformity and associated abnormalities. In: Ellis M, ed. *Modern trends in disease of the ear, nose and throat*. London: Butterworth, 1972; 219.
3. Satir P. How cilia move. *Scientific American* 1974; **231**: 45.
4. Drettner B, Aust R. Plethysmographic studies of the blood flow in the mucosa of the human maxillary sinus. *Acta Oto-laryngologica* 1974; **78**: 259.
5. Angaard A. Capillary and shunt blood flow in the nasal mucosa of cats. *Acta Oto-laryngologica 1974*; **78**: 419.
6. Arbour P, Kern EB. Paradoxical nasal obstruction. *Can J Otolaryngol* 1975; **4**: 333.
7. Burrows A, Eccles R. Reciprocal changes in nasal resistance to airflow caused by pressure applied to the axilla. *Acta Oto-laryngologica* 1985; **99**: 154.
8. Watson-Williams E. Endocrines and the nose. *J Laryngol Otol* 1952; **66**: 29.

Chapter 3

THE IMMUNOPHARMACOLOGY OF RHINITIS

P. H. Howarth

INTRODUCTION

The National Morbidity surveys from the Royal College of General Practitioners Unit in Birmingham, UK, have identified a quadrupling of the number of consultations for seasonal allergic rhinitis between the years of 1955/56 and 1980/81. While a number of factors may account for this, a diagnostic change is unlikely, as the classical constellation of acute rhinitic symptoms on exposure to an allergen to which an individual is sensitised is easily recognised, with nasal itching, sneezing, rhinorrhoea and transient nasal blockage. These immediate symptoms are a consequence of mast cell degranulation and the local release of inflammatory mediators. Involvement of mast cells in the immediate response has been demonstrated both indirectly, with evidence of local mast cell mediator release, and directly by the identification of allergen-related mast cell degranulation on nasal biopsy. Prolonged allergen exposure to a relevant allergen, as in perennial allergic rhinitis, reproduces these symptoms with nasal blockage often becoming a more prominent feature. The role of the mast cell or the other metachromatic staining cell, the basophil, in the persistence of nasal symptoms and their relevance to the secretory eosinophilia identified in these patients has yet to be fully clarified.

THE MAST CELL

The mast cell was first described in 1877 by Paul Ehrlich, when investigating the histochemical staining characteristics of some synthetic basic anilene dyes. He identified the presence of a connective tissue cell whose granules altered the colour of the dye (metachromasia). As these cells were numerous in connective tissue whose nutrition was enhanced, he named them mastzellen (well nourished cells).

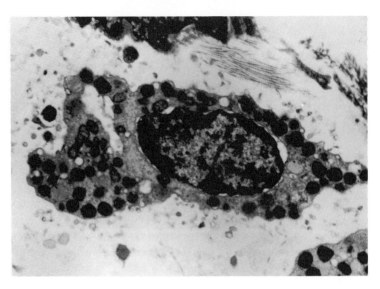

Figure 1a: Electron micrograph of human mast cell magnification ×16 000

Granular contents

Electron microscopy of a quiescent mast cell identifies a cytoplasm full of defined secretory granules. It is the high content of proteoglycan within these granules that confers the metachromatic staining characteristic, a property shared only with basophils. In human mast cells this proteoglycan is a 60kD species of heparin whose highly sulphated glycosaminoglycan (GAG) groups combine with the predominant proteases, tryptase, chymase or carboxypeptidase to form the characteristic crystalline structure of the granules (Fig. 1). Four structures of crystal have been described, scrolls, lattices, gratings and a serpentine-like structure, all of which have a common repeating periodicity of 7.5pm or multiples thereof, suggesting a similar basic chemical structure [1]. In addition to storing these potent proteolytic enzymes, heparin, at the acid pH within the secretory granules, also stores the basic amine histamine through simple ionic binding. These three granular components, histamine, heparin and the neutral proteases comprise the major pre-formed mediators of human mast cells. In addition smaller quantities (on a weight basis) of exoglycosidases, chemotactic factors (eosinophil and neutrophil), oxidative enzymes and a kininogenase have been described in association with human mast cells.

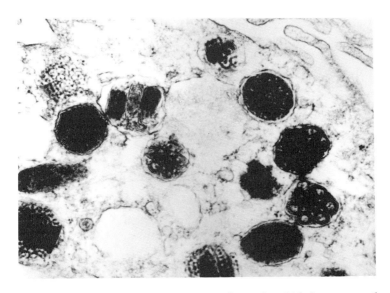

Figure 1b: Electron micrograph of human mast cell granules which demonstrates the characteristic crystalline structure magnification ×48 000

Immunoglobulin E

The crucial link between the mast cell and the immediate allergic reaction is immunoglobulin E (IgE). Immunoglobulin E, following its isolation in 1966 from the sera of ragweed-sensitive subjects, was identified as being the agent responsible for the transmission of the immediate hypersensitivity response [2], an action previously attributed to an unidentified "reaginic antibody". Immunoglobulin E functions as a cell surface antibody, binding to cell surfaces. Two cell surface receptors are described, a high affinity Fc_I receptor and a low affinity Fc_{II} receptor. The high afinity Fc_I receptors are present on human mast cells and basophils, with these cells possessing approximately 300 000 and 40 000–100 000 such receptors respectively [3]. The more recently described Fc_{II} receptors are present in lower numbers on macrophages, eosinophils, platelets and lymphocytes [4]. In the atopic state, in which there is a propensity for the excessive production of IgE to environmental allergens, IgE binds to Ige Fc receptors on mast cell surfaces. These sensitised cells are thus primed to react to specific environmental allergens. Exposure to the relevant allergen leads to cross linking of the surface IgE molecules which brings the high affinity IgE-Fc_I receptors into apposition and initiates a series of membrane and cytoplasmic events culminating in the release of the granule-associated, pre-formed mediators and the *de novo* synthesis of newly generated mediators. Enhanced IgE production also occurs in conditions associated with diminished T-lymphocyte suppressor cell activity, as in the primary immunodeficiency syndromes, such as the Wiskott-Aldrich syndrome and ataxia-telangectasia, and in acquired immunodeficiency states such as transient hypo-gamma-globulinaemia in children and some forms of lymphoma (eg Hodgkin's). These conditions may also be associated with symptoms characteristic of the atopic state.

MAST CELL ACTIVATION/SECRETION

Following immunological activation, there is an increase in intracellular calcium, solubulisation of the mast cell granules, movement of the granules by cytoskeletal proteins into apposition with the cell membrane, fusion of the perigranular and cytoplasmic membranes and liberation of the granule contents into the extracellular environment (Fig. 2). This process involves the activation of the phosphatidyl inositol (PI)—diacyl glycerol (DAG) pathway and the production of inositol triphosphate. Phosphatidyl inositol is a membrane phospholipid from which DAG is cleaved following cell activation, either by phospholipase C or after sequential methylation of PI by a phosphodiesterase [5]. Subsequent metabolism of DAG by the calcium-dependent enzyme diglyceride lipase leads not only to the production of L-monoacyl glycerol (MAG) but also arachidonic acid. The products of this pathway regulate intracellular events. Both DAG and MAG are potent membrane fusagens. In addition DAG activates the calcium-dependent enzyme protein kinase C which is responsible for the conversion of myosin to its active phosphorylated form, and hence induces contraction of smooth muscle (in this instance the contraction of the cytoskeletal thin filaments), leading to the movement of the granules towards the cell plasma membrane. Inositol triphosphate, formed during generation of DAG, can mobilise calcium from intracellular stores in the presence of ATP, making it available for calcium dependent enzymes. In addition to these intracellular changes, cell activation is accompanied by a transient increase in cellular levels of cyclic AMP which precedes mediator secretion.

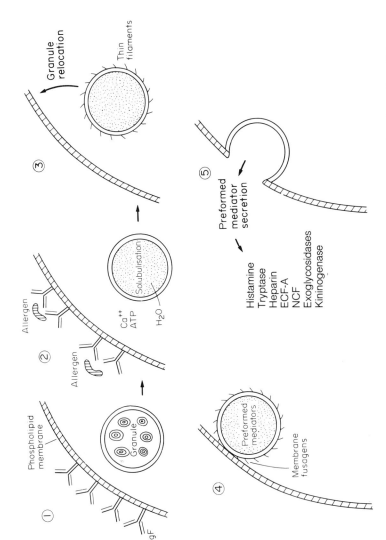

Figure 2: Sequence of immunological mast cell degranulation with secretion of preformed mediators.

37

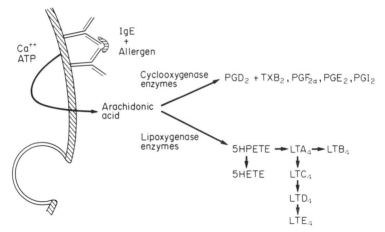

Figure 3: Production of newly generated mast cell mediators.

Newly generated mediators

The cleavage of arachidonic acid from the phospholipid membrane, following mast cell activation, is likely to involve primarily the phospholipase C/diglyceride lipase pathway as described, rather than the steroid-sensitive phospholipase A_2 pathway pertinent to some other cell types. The mobilised arachidonic acid is then metabolised by either cyclooxygenase enzymes to prostaglandins (PGs) and thromboxanes (TXs) or by lipoxygenase enzymes to hydroxyeicosatetranoeic acids (HETEs) and leukotrienes (LTs). Immunological stimulation of purified mast cells produces predominantly PGD_2 as the major prostanoid, with only small quantities of TXB_2, PGF_{2a}, PGE_2 and 6-keto-PGF_{1a} being produced [6]. In addition to generating prostanoids, activation of human mast cells is associated with generation of 5HETE, LTB_4, LTC_4 and to a lesser extent LTD_4 (Fig. 3). There is little evidence for human mast cells as being a major source of platelet activating factor (PAF) [7].

Mediator relevance *in vivo*

An understanding of the mediators and their secretory processes is only of relevance if this can be directly related to the disease under consideration. With respect to allergic rhinitis, it is possible to explain many of the features of this disease on the basis of mast cell mediator release (Fig. 4). Histamine nasal insufflation produces itching, sneezing, rhinorrhoea and transient nasal blockage [8]. These effects are predominantly mediated via H_1-receptors with only a small contribution to nasal blockage being related to vascular H_2-receptors. The hypersecretion is bilateral following unilateral nasal challenge, while the blockage is only on the challenged side. The bilateral hypersecretion is related to H_1-stimulation of sensory nerve endings with reflex parasympathetic activity to contralateral nasal glands.

In clinical practice, H_1-antihistamines reduce seasonally related sneezing and rhinorrhoea but have little effect on nasal blockage [9], suggesting that non-histamine mediators are of greater importance in the everyday genesis of this symptom. Possible contributors to nasal blockage are LTC_4, LTD_4 and PGD_2. Both LTC_4 and LTD_4 produce a dose-dependent sustained nasal blockage and an increase in nasal secretions with local application, in the absence of itching or sneezing [10, 11]. PGD_2 infusion in man is reported to be associated with "nasal stuffiness" consistent with the known vasodilator properties of this prostanoid. The interraction between histamine, PGD_2, PGI_2, PGE_2, LTC_4, LTD_4 which vasodilate, and LTC_4, LTD_4 and histamine, all of which enhance vascular permeability will lead to local fluid extravasation and tissue oedema, further compromising nasal airflow. These effects on nasal blockage could be compounded further by the chemoattractant properties of eosinophil chemotactic factor (ECF) and the more potent LTB_4, attracting eosinophils into tissue and mucosal sites. Eosinophils also possess IgE-receptors, of lower affinity than mast cells, and if immunologically activated would elaborate the inflammatory response, being able to synthesise the sulphidopeptide leukotrienes, to degranulate mast cells and to produce ciliary motility abnormalities impairing clearance of nasal secretions [12].

THE MAST CELL *IN VIVO*

Indirect approach

Lavage of the nasal cavity following intranasal allergen installation in sensitised subjects has been used to detect the local release mediators [13]. During the immediate nasal response to allergen installation there is an increase in histamine, PGD_2, LTC_4, LTD_4,

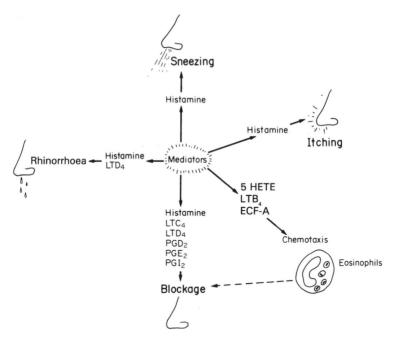

Figure 4: Inflammatory mediators in the genesis of rhinitic symptoms.

kinins and TAME esterase. While a number of these mediators could have other cell sources, their appearance in conjunction with PGD_2 would support a mast cell origin.

A number of patients also develop a late nasal obstructive response following allergen nasal challenge. Measurement of mediator release during the late response identifies elevations in histamine, kinins, LTC_4 and TAME esterase [14]. There is no apparent elevation in PGD_2. Short-term corticosteroid therapy (< 48 hours) inhibits both the obstruction and mediator release occurring during the late nasal response to allergen challenge but has no effect on the immediate response [15]. As glucocorticoids inhibit basophil but not mast cell degranulation *in vitro* and PGD_2 is mast cell and not basophil derived, this has led to the hypothesis that the basophil and not the mast cell is important in the late nasal obstructive response. By analogy with the relationship between the late phase airway response to allergen and clinical asthma, it has been suggested that the basophil (which also possesses high affinity, high density IgE receptors) is of greater relevance to perennial allergic rhinitis than the mast cell.

Direct approach

Direct evidence for mast cell degranulation following allergen nasal challenge has been investigated in nasal biopsy specimens. During the immediate nasal response substantial mast cell degranulation has been identified [16]. During the late nasal obstructive response an increase in secretory eosinophils, neutrophils and basophils but not mast cells is described [17].

Direct evidence for mast cell involvement has also been investigated in the clinical context. During natural seasonal exposure in grass pollen or birch pollen sensitive subjects there is an increase in metachromatic staining cells in the nasal mucosa [18]. Sequential biopsies show a migration of mast cells from the lamina propria to the mucosal surface and a total increase in mast cell numbers [18]. These newer mucosal metachromatic cells do not exhibit the classical staining properties of mast cells and may have differing morphological characteristics. These have been referred to as basophil or "basophiloid-like" cells. Similar metachromatic cells have been described in nasal smears, epithelial scrapings and mucosal sections in allergic nasal conditions, their number being in direct relationship with the clinical disease activity [19]. This differentiation between basophils and mast cells may be a reflection of cellular heterogeneity, in response to local stimuli rather than representing separate cell populations of distinctly different lineage. It is now realised that mast cells are not a homogeneous population.

MAST CELL HETEROGENEITY

The concept of mast cell heterogeneity was first described from rodent cells [20]. In these animals there are two major mast cell populations based on cell size, number of secretory granules, histamine content, secretory characteristics and histochemical fixation and staining properties. Of these the connective tissue mast cell is larger and contains more histamine than the mucosal mast cell. It is the latter which has been shown to proliferate during parasitic infection or following allergen sensitisation under the regulation of cytokines, including interleukin-3, secreted from activated T-lymphocytes.

It is therefore tempting to extrapolate these findings to the nose and liken the "basophiloid-like" cells, which increase on mucosal surfaces in response to allergen exposure, to the rodent mucosal mast cell, the standard staining technique being based on the connective tissue mast cell. In support of this is the identification of a proliferation of formaldehyde-sensitive mast cells throughout the pollen season in patients with allergic rhinitis and the inhibition of their appearance by regular corticosteroid therapy [21]. The availability of monoclonal and polyclonal antibodies to the mast cell proteases tryptase and chymase should now permit a more definitive appraisal of nasal mast cell heterogeneity. It has been shown in human lung and intestinal tissue that the proportion of tryptase and chymase within cells and the dependence of these cells upon T-derived maturation factors varies depending upon their location in relationship to the mucosal surface.

INVOLVEMENT OF OTHER CELL TYPES

It is apparent from the foregoing discussion that cells other than mast cells participate in the pathogenesis of rhinitis. Their exact involvement and their relationship to the mast cell has yet to be fully unravelled. The role of the basophil has already been discussed, in relationship to the late nasal response and to clinical disease. Considerable interest also centres on the eosinophil, a cell known to possess IgE receptors and to be activated on immunological challenge. This cell is identified in nasal smears from patients with non-infective rhinitis, not all of whom, apparently, have an allergic basis for their disease. Its granules contain eosinophil peroxidase (EPO) and major basic protein (MBP) which are both capable of degranulating mast cells [11]. MBP has in addition a potential for disrupting cilial and epithelial function, an effect apparent on ciliated human nasal epithelial cells *in vitro* but not apparent in the nose in seasonal allergic rhinitis [22]. The end organ effect of eosinophil derived newly generated mediators is uncertain, as both LTD_4 and PAF are produced, each having opposing actions. LTD_4 causes nasal blockage [10] while PAF reduces nasal resistance by decreasing mucosal blood flow and constricting venous capacitance vessels [23]. Other cells identified within nasal tissue following allergen exposure are monocytes and lymphocytes. Both these cell types possess low affinity IgE receptors and are likely to be involved in immune responses [4]. Indeed it is possible that interleukin-5 produced by lymphocytes is one of the major chemotactic stimuli for eosinophil accumulation. The interrelationship between these different cell lines is thus complex, a situation not clarified by the realisation that non-immunological mechanisms may also lead to mast cell activation with mediator release.

NON-IMMUNOLOGICAL MAST CELL SECRETAGOGUES

Non-immunological stimuli inducing mast cell degranulation, in addition to eosinophil derived products, include the complement components C3a and C5a, bacterial cell wall lectins, the neuropeptide substance P, the presence of a hyperosmolar environment and histamine releasing factors (HRF) [5]. The mechanism of mediator release with these agents is distinct from IgE orchestrated release. It is relevant to note, however, that interleukin-3 (IL-3) and granulocyte colony stimulating factor (G-CSF), both HRF in their own right, potentiate IgE-mediated histamine release when present in concentrations too low to promote secretion themselves [24]. Substance P-containing nerves are present in the nasal mucosa in a perivascular, periglandular and epithelial distribution. Nasal insufflation with substance P in man causes nasal blockage, facial flushing and tachycardia, identifying a systemic as well as a local effect [25]. This could be due to a direct effect of substance P on vessels but may alternatively be related to substance P-induced histamine release, which occurs in the absence of the generation of PGD_2 or LTC_4 [26].

THERAPEUTIC IMPLICATIONS

Although an allergic basis for rhinitis in atopic individuals is undisputed, avoidance of relevant allergens such as grass pollen or birch pollen in seasonal allergic disease is not practical without major modifications to lifestyle. A reduction in house dust exposure, however, through standard mite control procedures coupled with the use of acaricidals can significantly reduce house dust mite colonies with symptomatic benefit. Simple mite control measures in mite sensitive rhinitis (as detailed in Chapter 8) should therefore be standard before considering therapeutic intervention. Similarly a search for other relevant allergens, such as household pets, may be pertinent in some individuals.

Allergy testing

The relevance of an environmental allergen to rhinitis is often apparent from the history of either symptoms on specific exposure or with a characteristic seasonal periodicity. This can be confirmed by testing for the presence of IgE either bound to cutaneous mast cells (skin tests), or free in the circulation (RAST). Due to their simplicity, rapidity of performance, low cost and high sensitivity, skin tests remain a corner stone of allergy testing. They can be done either by intradermal administration of allergen or by epidermal prick or scratch testing. Of these, skin-prick testing (SPT) is most commonly employed as it is easy to perform, is virtually free from adverse effects, has a clearly discernible negative and positive response, is repeatable (especially with the recently introduced Morrow-Brown, stallerpointe or allergy-prick lancets which standardise the depth of penetration) and is acceptable in children. Intradermal testing (IDR) is disadvantageous in comparison with SPT as it (1) has a higher false positive response, (2) is painful and (3) may be associated on occasions with systemic reactions. If testing extracts of low allergenicity, however, IDR testing may offer advantages over standard SPT as it is a more sensitive method. Scratch testing has now been largely discontinued as it introduces a variable quantity of allergen.

The need for an alternative method other than SPT is due to the limitations of this method when testing patients with dermatographism or with extensive atopic dermatitis. The responses are unreliable in these conditions and the responses are also reduced in patients receiving H_1-antihistamines. In these circumstances measurement of specific circulating IgE by the radioallergosorbent test (RAST) offers an alternative diagnostic method. RAST correlates closely with SPT. It is an immunometric "sandwich"-type immunoassay in which excess amounts of allergen are attached to a solid phase. After the patient's serum is incubated with a solid phase allergen, the amount of allergen-specific IgE in the serum is quantified by incubation with radiolabelled anti-IgE. More recently, the radioactive labels used in earlier RAST assays have been replaced with enzyme labels that generate colour or fluorescence. A number of systems now offer a panel of different allergens that can be tested from one serum sample [27]. These systems are, however, expensive compared with skin-prick testing.

Pharmacotherapy

With respect to pharmacotherapy, H_1-antihistamines and corticosteroids still remain the main therapeutic agents for allergic

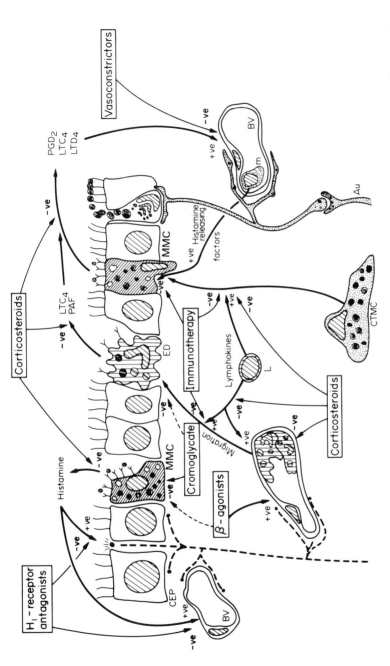

Figure 5: Sites of action of treatments for rhinitis. CEP=ciliated epithelial cells; MMC=mucosal metachromatic staining cell (mast cell or basophil); CTMC=connective tissue mast cell; EO=eosinophil; BV=blood vessel; M=monocytes; SNF=sensory nerve fibre; Au=autonomic efferent nerves; L=lymphocyte.

45

rhinitis (Fig.5). Histamine, whether mast cell or basophil derived, whether immunologically released or released as a consequence of mast cell activation by neuropeptides, eosinophil products, cell derived histamine releasing factors or local osmotic changes will have the same symptomatic effects, producing itching, sneezing and rhinorrhoea. Treatment with H_1-antihistamines reduces all these symptoms in both seasonal and perennial allergic rhinitis. Symptoms are not, however, abolished and there is little effect on nasal blockage with this form of therapy [9]. Despite this, H_1-antihistamines remain the most appropriate therapy for patients with transient and intermittent symptoms, in whom the immediate mast cell response is of prime importance. Additional or alternative treatment may be required in patients with more persistent symptoms.

As mediators other than histamine are important in allergic rhinitis and it is not possible to antagonise all their end organ effects, treatment has been directed at inhibiting cell activation to prevent mediator release. In respect to mast cells, both beta-agonists and cromoglycate-like drugs possess this action [28]. Beta-agonists, by raising intracellular cyclic AMP, inhibit immunologically stimulated mast cell mediator release, and are several thousand times more potent in this respect than cromoglycate, according to one *in vitro* study employing human lung mast cells [29]. Although intranasal administration of fenoterol, a beta$_2$-selective agonist, reduces the immediate laboratory response to allergen challenge [30], it has proved disappointing in clinical practice. This may be due to a vasodilator effect limiting its efficacy by increasing nasal resistance, or to pharmacological heterogeneity of the mucosal metachromatic cell. While beta-agonists are effective on mast cells they have little effect on immunologically-mediated basophil degranulation.

Cromoglycate-like drugs are thought to inhibit mast cell degranulation through actions on either protein kinase C [31] or through phosphorylation of a 78kD protein [32], both effects being associated with an interruption of the intracellular activation process. Like beta-agonists, these drugs overall have proved disappointing, tending to be more effective in limiting sneezing and runny nose than nasal blockage. The relevance of the discovery that cromoglycate has a differential effect on newly generated mediator release as compared to preformed mediator release from stimulated mast cells is difficult to put into this perspective. One report demonstrates an 85% reduction in PGD_2 release but only a 25% reduction in histamine release following immunological mast cell stimulation in the presence of cromoglycate [29]. A further possible limiting factor with cromoglycate therapy is the lack of effect of this drug on basophil degranulation. The newer cromoglycate-like drug, nedocromil, is more potent than cromoglycate in inhibiting immunological mast cell degranulation and has additional effects on eosinophil and neutrophil activation. Preliminary results with this agent suggest beneficial effects in the treatment of seasonal allergic rhinitis, although again with less of an effect on nasal blockage than on sneezing and rhinorrhoea.

Corticosteroids remain the most effective treatment for allergic rhinitis, reducing all symptoms including nasal blockage. They are known to have several modes of action of possible relevance: they influence eosinophil function, reducing both cell activation, through inhibiting production of lymphokines and monokines involved in the activation process, and total circulating eosinophil numbers. The eosinopenia following systemic corticosteroid administration may be related both to the cell margination on the intravascular endothelial surface limiting their chemotaxis, and to suppression of bone marrow production. Intranasal corticosteroid therapy inhibits the eosinophil accumulation in the nasal secretions in the late nasal response and in clinical practice reduces nasal eosinophil accumulation. Corticosteroids are also known to stimulate the production of an intracellular protein, lipomodulin, which inhibits phospholipase A_2, an enzyme involved in arachidonic acid cleavage [33]. Support for the phospholipase C/diglyceride lipase pathway for arachidonic acid cleavage in mast cell activation, is the failure of corticosteroids to have any influence on mast cell activation *in vitro*. Consistent with this is the failure of short-term corticosteroids to inhibit the immediate nasal response to allergen challenge. Corticosteroids do, however, inhibit the release of histamine, kinins, and TAME-esterase, and the accumulation of eosinophils within the nasal mucosa during the late nasal response to allergen challenge and are effective inhibitors of immunologically related basophil degranulation. Of further interest is the discovery that long term therapy with inhaled but not oral corticosteroid therapy inhibits the early response to allergen challenge within the nose. A clue to the mechanism of this action, and highlighting the importance of the mode of therapy, is the finding that inhaled corticosteroids inhibit the seasonally related migration of mast cells into the nasal mucosa, thereby limiting any allergen/ antibody interraction relevant to the immediate response [21]. This effect may be related to inhibition of lymphokine production by T-lymphocytes.

Other potential modes of therapy currently under clinical evaluation are the dipeptide, N-acetyl-aspartyl-glutamic acid (magnesium sulphate) (NAAGA) and the pentapeptide (HEPP), a synthetic peptide derived from the Fc region of human IgE. NAAGA is a naturally occurring brain dipeptide with a high affinity for glutamate receptors. It has been shown experimentally to (1) prevent anaphylactic and non-anaphylactic mast cell degranulation, (2) to inhibit both the cytolytic effect of the activated complement and the generation of anaphylotoxins, and (3) to attenuate allergen-induced nasal blockage in the laboratory [34]. HEPP has been more extensively investigated, inhibiting both experimentally-induced and naturally occurring sneezing, rhinorrhoea and nasal blockage in allergic rhinitis when administered either subcutaneously or intranasally [35]. The mechanism of action of HEPP is still under evaluation as it does not act by competing for native IgE on Fc receptors on mast cells and basophils as originally proposed.

Immunotherapy

Immunotherapy involves administering increasing concentrations of allergen extracts, to which a patient is sensitive, in an attempt to ameliorate the associated symptomatology through modulation of the immune response. This is usually administered subcutaneously, but oral and nasal routes of administration have been explored. Its introduction in 1911 was based on the assumption that it would work as for immunisation, through the stimulation of protective antibodies, before the relevance of IgE to symptom generation was appreciated. Despite its widespread use from this date, it was not until 1954 that a placebo-controlled study identified efficacy in the treatment of allergic rhinitis [36]. The mode of action of immunotherapy was initially considered to be due to the production of a "blocking antibody" of the IgG sub-class, but this is now not considered a major mechanism of action in inhalant allergy. More recently immunotherapy has been found to reduce the mediator secretion during the immediate nasal response to allergen challenge *in vivo*, this effect correlating with individual efficacy of treatment [37]. *In vitro* studies have identified a decreased sensitivity of basophils to allergen stimulation after immunotherapy, an effect possibly due to cytokines as during pollen immunotherapy mononuclear cells synthesise less histamine releasing factor [38]. Immunotherapy (like corticosteroids) has also been reported to reduce the number of metachromatic staining cells (mast cells and basophils) and eosinophils in the nasal mucosa in allergic rhinitis [39, 40], possibly through regulation of T-lymphocyte activity (Fig. 5).

CONCLUSION

Despite the increase in information concerning the immunology of rhinitis, the majority of this has centred on the immediate response and the mast cell. The relevance of this cell to the persistence of symptoms and its interraction with other cell types, now realised to be of relevance to symptom generation, has yet to be clarified. Further research directed towards an understanding of factors regulating local cell accumulation, cell maturation and cell activation within the nose is required to clarify these points. In addition, an understanding of mast cell maturation during migration and the influence on this process of pharmacological and immunotherapeutic agents is required to define therapeutic approaches and to determine if the circulating basophil serves as a better model for therapeutic effects within the nose than the present *in vitro* animal or human mast cell systems. In the current state of knowledge topical corticosteroid therapy which inhibits both mast cell and eosinophil accumulation and eosinophil and basophil activation within the nose is the most consistently effective treatment.

REFERENCES

1. Caulfield JP, Lewis RA, Hein A, Austen KF. Secretion of dissociated human pulmonary mast cells. Evidence for solubilization of granule contents before discharge. *J Cell Biol* 1980; **85**: 299-311.
2. Ishizaka K, Ishizaka T, Hornbrook MM. Physicochemical properties of human reaginic antibody. IV. Presence of a unique immunoglobulin as a carrier of reaginic activity. *J Immunol* 1966; **97**: 75-85.
3. Ishizaka T, Conrad DH. Binding characteristics of human IgE receptors and initial triggering events in human mast cells for histamine release. *Monogr Allergy* 1983; **18**: 14-24.
4. Capron A, Dessaint J-P, Tonnel AB. IgE receptors on inflammatory cells. In: Michel FB, Bousquet J, Goddard PH, [eds]. *Highlights in asthmology*. Berlin: Springer-Verlag 1987; 107-16.
5. Benyon RC. Stimulus-secretion coupling in mast cells and basophils. In: Holgate ST, ed. *Mast cells, mediators and disease*. Dordrecht: Kluwer 1988; 195-226.

6. Lewis RA, Soter NA, Diamond PT, Austen KF, Oates JA and Roberts LJ. Prostaglandin D_2 generation after activation of rat and human mast cells with anti-IgE. *J Immunol* 1982; **129**: 1627-31.
7. Robinson C. Mast cells and newly generated lipid mediators. In: Holgate ST, ed. *Mast cells, mediators and disease*. Dordrecht: Kluwer 1988; 149-74.
8. Mygind N, Secher C, Kirkegaard J. Role of histamine and antihistamines in the nose. *Eur J Respir Dis* 1983; **64** (Suppl 128): 16-20.
9. Howarth PH, Holgate ST. Comparative trial of two non-sedative H_1-antihistamines, terfenadine and astemizole, for hayfever. *Thorax* 1984; **39**: 668-72.
10. Bisgaard H, Olsson P, Bende M. Leukotriene D_4 increases nasal blood flow in humans. *Prostaglandins* 1984; **27**: 599-604.
11. Miadonna A, Tedeschi A, Leggiere E, Lorini M, Folco G, Sala A, Qualizza R, Froldi M, Zanussi C. Behaviour and clinical relevance of histamine and leukotrienes C_4 and B_4 in grass pollen-induced rhinitis. *Am Rev Resp Dis* 1987; **136**: 357-62.
12. Frigas E, Gleich GJ. The role of eosinophils in allergy. In: Lessof M H, Lee T H, Kemeny D M, eds. *Allergy: An international textbook*, Chichester: Wiley 1987: 137-55.
13. Naclerio RM, Meier H L, Kagey-Sobotka, *et al*. Mediator release after nasal airway challenge with allergen. *Am Rev Resp Dis* 1983; **128**: 597-602.
14. Naclerio RM, Togias RG, Proud D, *et al*. Inflammatory mediators in late antigen-induced rhinitis. *N Engl J Med* 1985; **313**: 65-70.
15. Mygind N, Johnson NJ, Thomsen J. Intranasal allergen challenge during corticosteroid treatment. *Clin Allergy* 1977; **7**: 69.
16. Corrado OJ, Gomez E, Baldwin DL, Swanston AR, Davies RJ. Direct evidence for mast cell involvement in type I allergic reactions in man. *Thorax* 1985; **40**: 218.
17. Pipkorn U. Hayfever: in the laboratory and at natural allergen exposure. *Allergy* 1988; **43** (Suppl 8): 41-4.
18. Enerback L, Granerus G, Pipkorn U. Intraepithelial migration of mast cells in hayfever. *Int Arch Allergy Appl Immunol* 1986; **80** : 44-54.
19. Otsuka H, Denburg JA, Dolovich J, *et al*. Heterogeneity of metachromatic cells in human nose: significance of mucosal mast cells. *J Allergy Clin Immunol* 1985; **76**: 695-702.
20. Enerback L. The gut mucosal mast cell. *Monogr Allergy* 1981; **17**: 222-32.
21. Otsuka H, Denburg JA, Befus AD, *et al*. Effect of beclomethasone diproprionate on nasal metachromatic cell sub-populations. *Clin Allergy* 1986; **16**: 589-96.
22. Davies RJ. Mast cells in the nose. *Proc BSACI*, Cambridge 1988: S7/1.
23. Pipkorn N, Karlsson G, Bake B. Effect of platelet activating factor on human nasal mucosa. *Allergy* 1984; **39**: 141-5.
24. Kaplan AP. Histamine releasing factors. *Proc BSACI*, Cambridge 1988: S1/4.
25. Malm L, Petersson G. Tachykinins and nasal secretion. In: Hakansson R, Sundler R, eds. *Tachykinin antagonists*, Amsterdam: Elsevier 1985.
26. Benyon RC, Robinson C, Church MK. Differential release of histamine and eicosanoids from human skin mast cells by IgE-dependent and non-immunological stimuli (in press).
27. Brown CR, Higgins KW, Frazer K, *et al*. Simultaneous determination of total IgE and allergen-specific IgE in serum by the MAST Chemiluminescent assay system. *Clin Chem* 1985; **31**: 1500-5.
28. Howarth PH, Durham SR, Lee TH, Kay AB, Church MK, Holgate ST. Influence of albuterol, cromolyn sodium and ipratroprium bromide on the airway and circulating mediator responses to antigen bronchial provocation in asthma. *Am Rev Resp Dis* 1985; **132**: 986-92.
29. Church MK, Hiroi J. Inhibition of IgE-dependent histamine release from human

dispersed lung mast cells by anti-allergic drugs and salbutamol. *Br J Pharmacol* 1987; **90**: 421-9.

30. Borum P, Mygind N, Larsen FS. The anti-allergic effect of the beta$_2$-adrenergic agent fenoterol in the nose. *Env J Resp Dis* 1983; **64** (Suppl 128): 44-8.

31. Sagi-Eisenberg R. Possible role for a calcium-activated phospholipid-dependent protein kinase in mode of action of DSCG. *Trends Pharmacol Sci* 1985; **6**: 198-200.

32. Theoharides TC, Seighart W, Greengard P, Douglas WW. Antiallergic drug cromolyn may inhibit secretion by regulating phosphorylation of a mast cell protein. *Science* 1980; **207**: 80-2.

33. Blackwell GJ, Carmiccio R, Di Rossa M, Flower RJ, Parente L, Persico P. Macrocortin: a polypeptide causing the anti-phospholipase effect of glucocorticoids. *Nature* 1980; **287**: 147-9.

34. Ghaem A. A preliminary evaluation of the effect of N-acetyl-aspartyl-gluta mate on pollen nasal challenge as measured by rhinomanometry and symptomatology. *Allergy* 1987; **42**: 626-30.

35. Prenner BM. Double-blind placebo controlled trial of intranasal IgE Pentapeptide. *Ann Allergy* 1987; **58**: 332-9.

36. Frankland AW, Angustin R. Prophylaxis of summer hay-fever and asthma: a controlled trial comparing crude grass-pollen extracts with the isolated main protein component. *Lancet* 1954; **i**: 1055-7.

37. Creticos PS, Adkinson NF, Kagey-Sobotka A, *et al*. Nasal challenge with ragweed pollen in hayfever patients. *J Clin Invest* 1985; **76**: 2247-53.

38. Malling H-J, Skov PS, Permin H, Norn S, Weeke B. Basophil histamine release and humoral changes during immunotherapy. Dissociation between basophil-bound specific IgE, serum values and cell sensitivity. *Allergy* 1982; **37**: 187-92.

39. Okuda M, Otsuka H. Basophil cells in allergic nasal secretions. *Arch Oto Rhino Laryngol* 1977; **214**: 85-9.

40. Rak S, Hakansson L, Venge P. Eosinophil chemotactic activity in allergic patients during the birch pollen season: the effect of immunotherapy. *Int Arch Allergy Appl Immunol* 1987; **82**: 349-50.

51

Chapter 4

RHINOMANOMETRY AND NASAL CHALLENGE

R. Eccles

NORMAL NASAL RESISTANCE

The nose acts as an air conditioning unit to warm, humidify and filter the inspired air. In order to mix and condition all the air effectively the airstream through the nasal passages must be turbulent. The changing direction and velocity of the inspired airstream ensure turbulent airflow but also provide a considerable resistance against respiratory airflow. When nasal breathing the nose contributes up to two-thirds of total respiratory resistance.

The narrowest point of the nasal passages determines the overall resistance to airflow and this region is often referred to as the "nasal valve". This region is situated at the anterior end of the inferior nasal turbinate just within the first few millimetres of the bony cavum and this is the site of maximum airway resistance and the narrowest point of the whole respiratory tract. The importance of the nasal valve region is illustrated in Fig. 1 which shows the changes in nasal resistance along the length of one nasal passage. The compliant nasal vestibule region contributes approximately one-third of nasal resistance and the nasal valve contributes nearly all of the remaining two-thirds of nasal resistance with only a very small contribution from the main turbinated region of the nasal passage.

In normal subjects the nasal resistance to airflow can vary with various factors such as exercise and posture and these factors will be discussed later. The changes in nasal resistance are determined by the state of engorgement of the inferior turbinate as when the blood vessels in the mucosa are congested the turbinate swells forward and can totally obstruct the airway. The anterior end of the inferior turbinate can advance by as much as 5mm when histamine is sprayed into the nose.

The level of congestion of blood vessels in the inferior turbinate regulates nasal resistance and there is little control over resistance

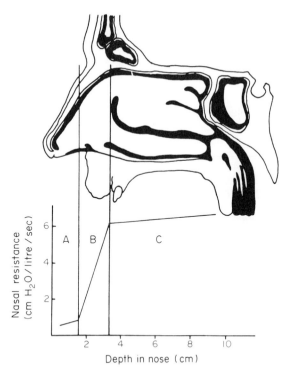

Figure 1: Changes in nasal resistance to airflow along a nasal passage. Approximately one-third of the resistance lies in the nasal vestibule and two-thirds just anterior to the inferior nasal turbinate at the level of the ''nasal valve''. (Based on the results of a study by Haight and Cole, 1983).

from the compliant nasal vestibule. On forced inspiration there is a tendency for the compliant walls of the nasal vestibule to collapse and limit airflow and this is normally prevented by contraction of the alae nasi muscles which splint or stabilise the alar wing of the nose and prevent collapse. The alae nasi muscles are activated whenever breathing is forced or distressed and flaring of the nostrils during inspiration is apparent during heavy exercise and in neonatal respiratory distress.

Normal nasal resistance in the adult is usually around 2–3 cm H_2O/l/sec and there is a gradual decrease in nasal resistance with increasing age. Nasal breathing is more comfortable than oral breathing as the mouth tends to dry and it is difficult to breathe through the mouth during sleep. The level of nasal resistance which would cause a subject to present with uncomfortable nasal obstruction is difficult to define as patients seem to be able to adapt with time to very high levels of nasal resistance and become obligatory mouth breathers. If one questions this group about their nasal breathing they often consider it to be normal, as over a period of years they have adapted to the situation of oral breathing. An acute nasal obstruction with nasal infection or allergy creates discomfort because the subject is aware of the change in nasal airflow and other nasal symptoms such as sneezing and runny nose, whereas a chronic condition of nasal obstruction, perhaps associated with a cleft palate or other developmental problem, does not create discomfort.

A ''normal'' nose is difficult to find in the population as in autumn and spring many subjects are either recovering from a common cold or developing one, and in spring and summer the hay fever season excludes another large group of the population. If one also excludes the subjects with perennial allergic rhinitis and those subjects with a deviated nasal septum then one is left with a very small group of ''normal'' noses.

Because the nose is at the entrance of the respiratory tract it is constantly exposed to infective and allergic insults and perhaps rather than being surprised at the high incidence of nasal disease we should expect even more problems, especially when one considers the very wide range of domestic and industrial environments that influence the physical and chemical properties of the air we breathe.

CONTROL OF NASAL RESISTANCE

Nasal resistance to airflow is primarily determined by the state of congestion of the blood vessels in the inferior turbinate and anterior nasal septum. An inspection of the histological appearance of the nasal mucosa in this region reveals that the tissue is erectile in nature with many venous sinusoids. As described above, this tissue can congest and swell and completely obstruct the nasal airway.

The level of congestion of the venous erectile tissue is primarily determined by the level of activity of the sympathetic vasoconstrictor nerves supplying the nasal blood vessels. Section of the cervical sympathetic nerve or local anaesthesia of the stellate sympathetic ganglion leads to Horner's syndrome with ipsilateral nasal congestion. This indicates that there is a constant sympathetic vasoconstrictor tone to the nasal erectile tissue and reduction of this sympathetic activity causes nasal congestion. Application of topical vasoconstrictor substances in nasal sprays mimics to some extent activation of the sympathetic nerves to the nasal blood vessels, as the nasal decongestant drugs are sympathomimetics.

Vasodilator substances such as histamine cause nasal congestion by filling the venous erectile tissue and this mechanism is probably the cause of nasal congestion in allergic rhinitis.

FACTORS THAT INFLUENCE NASAL RESISTANCE

Nasal resistance to airflow is influenced by many factors and some of the main factors are illustrated in Fig. 2 and discussed below.

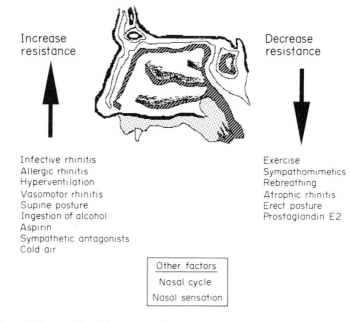

Increase
resistance

Decrease
resistance

Infective rhinitis
Allergic rhinitis
Hyperventilation
Vasomotor rhinitis
Supine posture
Ingestion of alcohol
Aspirin
Sympathetic antagonists
Cold air

Exercise
Sympathomimetics
Rebreathing
Atrophic rhinitis
Erect posture
Prostaglandin E2

Other factors

Nasal cycle

Nasal sensation

Figure 2: Factors that influence nasal resistance.

Nasal cycle

The airflow through the nasal passages is normally asymmetrical and most normal subjects show a regular cyclic change in nasal airflow as shown in Fig. 3. A nasal cycle is found in 80% of the population, yet most subjects are completely unaware of any changes in nasal airflow

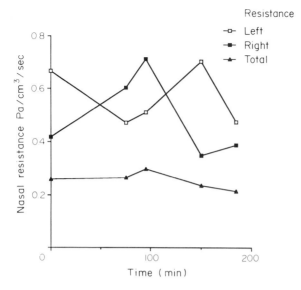

Figure 3: Cyclic changes in nasal airflow in a normal subject. The airflow through the right and left nasal passages varies in a reciprocal manner with the total resistance remaining more constant.

because the total resistance to airflow remains relatively constant due to a reciprocal relationship between the nasal passages.

The regular changes in nasal airflow are due to changes in sympathetic tone to the venous erectile tissue of the nasal mucosa with the low resistance side of the nose having the greatest sympathetic vasoconstrictor tone.

The nasal cycle appears to be regulated from the brainstem respiratory areas which control the activity of the sympathetic nerves to the nose. The functional significance of the cycle has not been satisfactorily explained. It is not just found in man but has also been described in the cat, rabbit, rat and pig. A simple explanation for the alternation in airflow would be that one side of the nose goes through a rest period and recovers from the minor traumas of conditioning the inspired air.

Exercise

Exercise is one of the most efficient ways of decongesting a blocked nose. On exercise there is a generalised increase in sympathetic vasoconstrictor tone to the nasal blood vessels and this causes a fall in nasal resistance to airflow. Exercise is a more potent nasal decongestant than topically applied vasoconstrictors since the increase in sympathetic vasoconstrictor tone affects all the nasal erectile tissue whereas the actions of a topical vasoconstrictor are limited to the site of application.

Respiration

Changes in the pattern of respiration can influence nasal resistance to airflow if they cause a change in arterial carbon dioxide. An increase in arterial carbon dioxide due to rebreathing or asphyxia causes a pronounced nasal vasoconstriction and a reduction in nasal resistance to airflow. In contrast hyperventilation causes nasal vasodilation and an increase in nasal resistance to airflow. These changes are due to reflex changes in sympathetic vasoconstrictor tone due to the effects of carbon dioxide on central and peripheral chemoreceptors.

Posture

Changes in posture can cause marked changes in nasal resistance to airflow due to changes in venous pressure and due to a skin pressure reflex.

The change from erect to supine posture causes an increase in total nasal resistance to airflow due to an increase in jugular venous pressure and an increased congestion of nasal venous erectile tissue.

On adoption of the lateral recumbent posture reflex changes in nasal resistance occur so that the dependent nasal passage congests and the upper nasal passage decongests. This partitioning of nasal airflow ensures that the upper nasal passage is responsible for the major component of nasal airflow and that the dependent nasal passage which could be obstructed by contact with the ground or pillow has little role in ventilation. The switching of airflow to the upper nasal passage overrides the partitioning of nasal airflow due to the nasal cycle. The changes in nasal airflow on adoption of the lateral recumbent posture are due to a skin pressure reflex with the axillary region being the most sensitive area for the initiation of the reflex.

Reciprocal changes in nasal airflow may be obtained by alternately lying on one side and then the other as shown in Fig. 4.

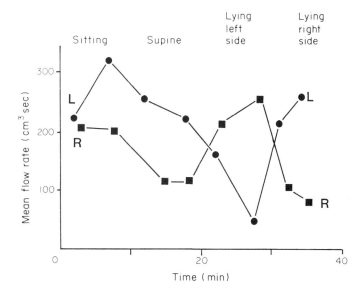

Figure 4: The effects of changes in posture on nasal airflow in one subject. Changing from lying on one side to the other caused reciprocal changes in nasal airflow.

Responses to thermal stimuli

The nasal blood vessels can be influenced by two kinds of thermal stimuli, changes in the temperature of the inspired air and changes in body skin temperature. Breathing cold air causes nasal congestion due to filling of venous erectile tissue and an increase in nasal resistance to airflow. In contrast the application of a cold stimulus to the skin causes nasal vasoconstriction but no change in nasal resistance to airflow. This indicates that cooling of the skin causes a reduction in nasal blood flow without any change in the volume of the venous erectile tissue. The reduction in nasal blood flow caused by cooling the skin may be useful in controlling epistaxis as many remedies recommend application of ice or a cold cloth to the skin.

Drugs

Ingestion of alcohol causes peripheral vasodilation and nasal congestion, especially when lying down. Aspirin has also been shown to cause nasal congestion. Drugs such as reserpine which antagonise the sympathetic nervous system in the treatment of hypertension cause nasal congestion. Prostaglandin E_2 has been shown to be a potent nasal vasoconstrictor with ten times the biological activity of adrenaline.

Sensation of airflow

The subjective sensation of airflow is very important as regards patient comfort but it is a parameter that is often overlooked by surgeons. The sensation of nasal airflow is provided by the cooling of sensory receptors in the nose on inspiration. These sensory receptors are supplied by the trigeminal nerve and anaesthesia or damage of the nerve causes a sensation of nasal obstruction. It is interesting that subjects with atrophic rhinitis often present with a complaint of nasal obstruction even though their nasal resistance to airflow is very low due to atrophy of nasal turbinates. In this disease the sensation of nasal obstruction is due to loss of sensation of nasal airflow.

Chronic nasal obstruction is often treated by surgical resection of turbinates or diathermy of mucosal tissue and both these procedures damage sensory nerve endings and can lead to a paradoxical sensation of nasal obstruction.

The sensation of nasal airflow is enhanced by aromatics such as menthol which are frequently incorporated in preparations used to treat nasal congestion associated with the common cold. Menthol sensitises nasal trigeminal sensory receptors and creates a sensation of improved airflow. There is also some evidence that menthol acts as a nasal decongestant and influences the activity of accessory respiratory muscles which stabilise the airway especially during sleep.

MEASUREMENT OF NASAL RESISTANCE AND RHINOMANOMETRY

As discussed above, the subjective sensation of nasal resistance to airflow can be very misleading and it is difficult to determine the level of nasal resistance by rhinoscopic examination except in extreme cases of obstruction or patency. In order to get a more objective measure of nasal resistance it is necessary to measure nasal pressure and flow parameters and calculate nasal resistance. Rhinomanometry is the term used to describe the measurement of nasal pressure and flow and the calculation of nasal resistance to airflow. Rhinomanometry is the most commonly used technique for measuring nasal resistance but there are several other methods such as determination of inspiratory peak nasal flow and acoustic rhinometry.

Rhinomanometry

Nasal resistance to airflow is calculated from measurements of nasal airflow and transnasal pressure. There is one pressure gradient across the nose which generates the airflows through the two nasal passages as shown in Fig. 5.

Many types of equipment are available for rhinomanometry but the basic method involves pressure and flow transducers connected to a microcomputer for data analysis and storage. A visual display of the pressure/flow relationship is essential in order to detect errors in measurement. A typical set of equipment is illustrated in Fig. 6.

The relationship between pressure and flow is complex due to turbulent airflow and a plot of pressure against flow is curvilinear as shown in Fig. 7. It is therefore necessary to define the point on the

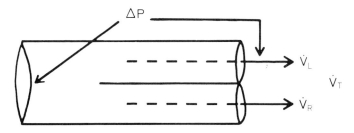

ΔP Pressure change across nose
$\dot{V}_L$ Left nasal airflow
$\dot{V}_R$ Right nasal airflow
$\dot{V}_T$ Total nasal airflow

Figure 5: Model of the nose to illustrate parameters measured in the determination of nasal resistance. The pressure gradient is from the posterior nares to the entrance of the nostril; this creates the airflows from the right and left nasal passages and the combined total nasal airflow.

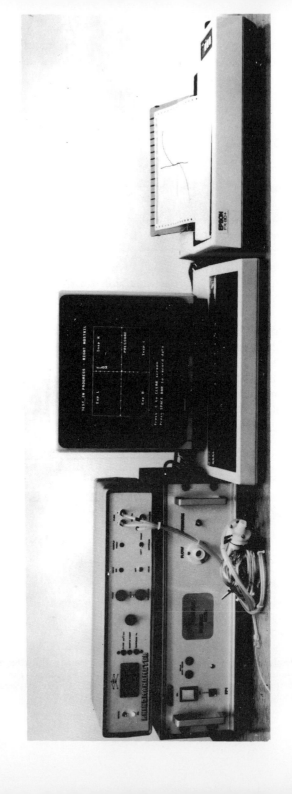

Figure 6: Equipment used to measure nasal resistance. From left to right, rhinomanometer (top) connected to face mask, flow and pressure calibrator (bottom), television display and microcomputer, printer. (Supplied by Mercury Electronics, Glasgow Ltd.)

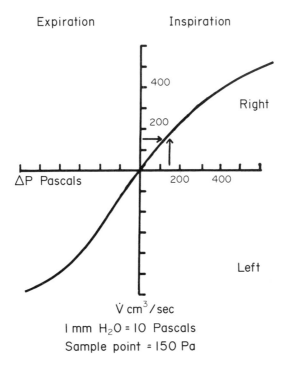

Expiration   Inspiration

ΔP Pascals

$\dot{V}$ cm^3/sec

I mm H$_2$O = IO Pascals

Sample point = I50 Pa

Figure 7: Typical x/y plot for nasal pressure and flow. In order to calculate nasal resistance the nasal airflow is measured at sample pressure of 150 Pa. Note that nasal resistance varies with the slope of the curve and therefore it is necessary to define the sample pressure point.

curve where resistance is measured and this is usually at a pressure of 150 Pa for anterior rhinomanometry.

Active anterior rhinomanometry involves measuring the pressure flow values of each nasal passage separately and then calculating the total resistance as shown in Fig. 8. Active posterior rhinomanometry measures both nasal passages simultaneously as shown in Fig. 9. The term "active" implies that the subject is breathing normally and generating the pressure and flow gradients through the nose by respiratory movements in contrast to passive rhinomanometry where the air is blown through the nose.

In all the above methods of rhinomanometry the resistance is calculated by dividing the pressure gradient by the flow and expressing resistance in units of pressure and flow.

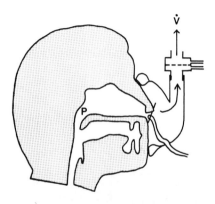

Figure 8: Active anterior rhinomanometry. One nostril is sealed with a pressure sensing tube by means of surgical tape in order to measure posterior nares pressure. Nasal airflow is measured from the other nostril. Pressure and flow are measured with normal quiet breathing. Transnasal pressure is measured across the nasal passage from posterior nares to mask. The resistance to airflow of each nasal passage is measured separately by taping the pressure sensing cannula alternately from one nostril to the other. Anterior rhinomanometry cannot be used if one nasal passage is completely obstructed.

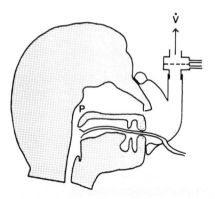

Figure 9: Active posterior rhinomanometry. Posterior nares pressure is sensed by means of an oral cannula. Total nasal airflow may be measured from both nostrils simultaneously or, by sealing one nostril at a time, the separate nasal airflows may be measured. Subjects require training to perform posterior rhinomanometry as there must be an airway between the oral and nasal cavities in order to sense the posterior nares pressure.

Nasal peak flow measurements

Expiratory peak flow gives a good measure of respiratory function in the treatment of asthma and it has the advantage of being a quick and cheap method of determining the level of bronchial obstruction.

Mini peak flow meters have been adapted for the measurement of nasal inspiratory peak flow and these have proved useful in measuring large changes in nasal resistance. The measurement of nasal peak flow is not as reproducible as the standard techniques of rhinomanometry but it does give a rough and ready guide to the level of nasal obstruction before and after nasal challenge.

Acoustic rhinometry

Acoustic rhinometry involves the measurement of a pressure wave reflected back from the nasal passage. The pressure wave is usually generated by a spark generator and the wave is directed towards the nose through a connecting tube. A microphone on the tube detects the pressure waves reflected back from the nasal passage and sends this signal for analysis. This method has the advantage that as well as calculating the resistance of the nasal passage it can also give an indication of the site of the narrowest region of the nasal passage.

NASAL CHALLENGE

Nasal challenge or nasal provocation tests involve the administration of suspected allergens directly into the nose in order to determine the nasal sensitivity of a test substance. In cases where there is some doubt over skin prick tests or blood RAST tests then direct nasal challenge may provide valuable diagnostic evidence of sensitivity.

Although nasal challenge tests have been used for research purposes their clinical usefulness remains to be evaluated. It has been claimed that allergy can be localised to the nose and be demonstrated by nasal challenge but not by skin or blood tests. Nasal challenge has been shown to be particularly useful in evaluating sensitivity to industrial and occupational allergens.

At present there is no standardised method of administering the test allergen or recording the response to the allergen. The method of administering an allergen varies from one centre to another with nasal drops, nebulized droplets, powders and allergen soaked filter paper discs all being used. The severity of the response to nasal challenge may be measured in terms of sneezes, secretion, nasal resistance, mediator levels or by measuring markers such as plasma proteins in nasal secretion. Measurement of one parameter such as nasal resistance is not satisfactory in determining the response to challenge as there is wide variation in the allergic symptoms between individuals, some subjects complaining mainly of sneezing and nasal irritation with not much congestion, and others complaining mainly of obstruction with little nasal irritation.

LOCAL AND REFLEX EFFECTS OF NASAL CHALLENGE

The nasal irritation, sneezing and hypersecretion caused by allergen challenge are due to stimulation of sensory nerves in the nasal mucosa. There is evidence that histamine is involved in these responses as they are reduced by H_1 histamine antagonists such as chlorpheniramine. From these studies it has been proposed that there are histamine H_1 receptors on the sensory nerves supplying the nasal mucosa.

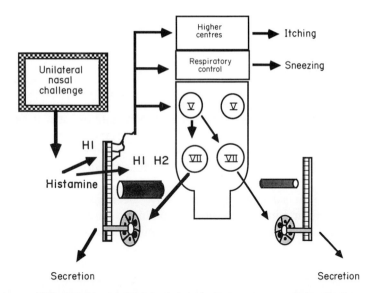

Figure 10: Diagram of responses to unilateral nasal challenge with histamine. The diagram shows the nasal mucosa, trigeminal sensory nerves, nasal blood vessels and glands, and the brainstem region. Histamine directly stimulates H_1 and H_2 receptors on nasal blood vessels to cause ipsilateral nasal congestion. Histamine also stimulates H_1 receptors on nasal sensory nerves and reflexly causes bilateral nasal secretion with the larger response ipsilateral to the challenge. The stimulation of sensory nerves by histamine also causes nasal itching and sneezing. (V) nucleus of trigeminal sensory nerves, (VII) nucleus of secretory area of seventh cranial nerve.

The nasal congestion caused by allergen challenge is due to the local vasodilator effects of mediators released from basophils. Unilateral nasal challenge causes bilateral nasal secretion but unilateral nasal congestion and this indicates that the secretion is induced reflexly by stimulation of sensory nerves and that the congestion is due to the local actions of the mediators, as shown in Fig. 10.

The allergic response in the nose is caused by a complex mixture of mediators whose time course of release and activation varies widely. Histamine release can explain many of the symptoms but recent studies indicate that kinins and prostaglandins may also have a significant role in the response. It is not therefore surprising that drugs directed solely against antagonising the effects of histamine can only provide partial relief from the allergic symptoms.

BIBLIOGRAPHY

Cole P. Nasal airflow resistance. In: Mathew OP, Sant'Ambrogio G, eds. *Respiratory function of the upper airway. Lung biology in health and disease*, volume 35, New York: Marcel Dekker, 1988: 391–414.

Eccles R. Rhinomanometry and nasal challenge. In: Mackay IS, Bull TR, eds. *Scott-Brown's Otolaryngology*, volume 4, *Rhinology*. London: Butterworth, 1987: 40–53.

Eccles R. Neurological and pharmacological considerations. In: Proctor DF, Andersen I, eds. *The nose: upper airway physiology and the atmospheric environment*. Amsterdam: Elsevier Biomedical, 1982: 191– 214.

Haight JSJ, Cole P. The site and function of the nasal valve. *The Laryngoscope* 1983; **93**: 49–55.

Chapter 5

OLFACTOMETRY AND THE SENSE OF SMELL

Victoria Moore-Gillon

INTRODUCTION

When doctors consider the reasons for treating rhinitis they tend to think purely in terms of nasal obstruction, and are prepared to offer a variety of methods for its relief. Rarely do they ask patients with rhinitis whether there is any disturbance of the sense of smell. If they were to ask, the patient's reply would in virtually every case be a slightly surprised "of course". To the individual with rhinitis, loss or impairment of the sense of smell is such an obvious accompaniment to the nasal obstruction that he or she assumes that the doctor must be aware of the problem.

Ignoring the sense of smell is almost universal amongst doctors in spite of the frequency with which olfactory disorders occur in the population. The degree of disruption to daily life that is experienced by the patient with reduced or absent smell is, of course, much less apparent than with major losses in the other senses and it is perhaps for this reason that the subject elicits little interest in clinicians. The patient, though, has problems quite apart from the obvious one of loss of enjoyment of everyday odours. There are often worries about inability to detect spoiled food, leaking gas and fire. Odour is a major component of what we usually think of as taste, and indeed in the majority of patients complaining of taste disorders, taste function itself is normal but there is unrecognised smell loss. Impairment of the sense of smell may be responsible for mood change, and there is an increased incidence of depression in people who become anosmic. There is some evidence linking olfactory impairment with sexual dysfunction, although this is still disputed by some authorities. Trivial though it may be to the doctor, smell is important to the patient.

In addition to a lack of awareness of the problem, one reason why smell has been ignored to such an extent is that there have, until recently, been no accurate and relatively simple ways of assessing olfaction. In the last decade, there have been advances both in understanding of basic olfactory physiology and in quantitatively testing the sense of smell in the clinical setting. There is now no reason why the success of any treatment for rhinitis should not be gauged by improvements in the sense of smell: why not use olfactometry rather than rhinomanometry? This may appear to be a rather revolutionary and iconoclastic suggestion, but if we are trying to measure improvement in the patient's symptoms then there is no more justification for using rhinomanometry alone than there is for using olfactometry alone.

When, in everyday life, we "smell" something we are usually not simply detecting impulses from the olfactory nerve. A more accurate—but inelegant—description of what is going on would be to refer to a "total odour experience". This experience is made up from input to the brain from the trigeminal, glossopharyngeal and vagus nerves, as well as the olfactory nerve. This fact can produce considerable difficulties during testing. A patient may have no true olfactory function at all, but may claim to be able to detect "strong smells" like ammonia or bleach. These substances, and many others, not only have a true odour but can also be detected by stimulation of trigeminal irritant receptors. True *odour* perception depends upon:-

1. The anatomical state of the nose.
2. The functional state of the olfactory epithelium.
3. The state of the peripheral and central nervous system.

Some understanding of the process of olfaction is thus essential if the pitfalls of olfactometry are to be avoided. This chapter will accordingly deal first with an outline of the relevant anatomy and physiology, and then go on to discuss the ways in which olfaction can be investigated and recorded.

ANATOMY AND PHYSIOLOGY OF OLFACTION

The olfactory epithelium occupies about 1 cm^2 on each side of the nose in the area of the cribriform plate and on the upper parts of the septum and superior turbinate. During normal quiet breathing, when the flow of air through the nose is low, only 5–10% of the inspired air reaches this area. Flow rates when sniffing are much

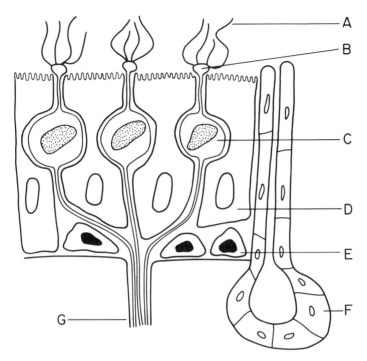

Figure 1: Schematic diagram of olfactory epithelium. A— cilia. B—dendritic knob. C—bipolar receptor neurone. D—supporting cell. E—basal cell. F—Bowman's gland. G—olfactory axon.

higher, and in addition the flow pattern changes so that 20% of this increased total flow reaches the olfactory epithelium. The epithelium is highly specialised and its structures are shown diagrammatically in Fig. 1. It is easily recognised under the electron microscope by the long cilia which project from the bipolar olfactory neurones. These cilia, unlike those elsewhere in the nose and respiratory tract, have no capacity for movement but instead are involved in odour reception and transduction.

The mechanisms by which odours are detected, transduced into olfactory nerve impulses, and recognised are only recently becoming clear. Odour molecules are carried to receptors on the cilia of olfactory neurones by a binding globulin which is present in the nasal mucus. These cilial receptors are glycoproteins and, much like antibodies, they probably have both fixed and variable regions, the latter selectively binding to different odour molecules. The binding of an odour molecule produces allosteric changes in the receptor

Table 1: *Nasal conditions associated with olfactory dysfunction*

Acute coryza
Allergic rhinitis
Vasomotor rhinitis
Sinusitis
Nasal polyposis
Septal deviation
Nasal and paranasal sinus tumours
Tumours of the nasopharynx
Granulomatous nasal conditions.

---

which activates a stimulatory GTP-binding protein. This in turn activates the enzyme adenyl cyclase and sets in motion a cascade of events resulting in ion conductance changes in the membrane and hence depolarisation.

Recent theories suggest that the cells are broadly "tuned": each neurone will respond to many odours, but no two neurones respond to exactly the same odours. Odours are thus recognised by the *combination* of olfactory neurones in which membrane depolarisation occurs. For any one odour, an individual and unique pattern of neuronal stimulation is produced, and it is this unique pattern of stimulation which gives rise to the characteristic olfactory sensation associated with that odour.

The last factor upon which odour perception depends is the state of the peripheral and central nervous system. The axons of the primary olfactory neurones pass through the cribriform plate to synapse in the olfactory bulb. The second order neurones are called mitral and tufted cells and their axons form the lateral olfactory tracts, which then project to the olfactory cortical regions in the temporal lobe. There is increasing interest in these pathways since we have come to realise that conditions such as Alzheimer's disease, Parkinson's disease, Huntington's chorea and Korsakoff's psychosis are associated with smell loss.

NASAL CONDITIONS ASSOCIATED WITH OLFACTORY LOSS

It is important to offer the patient with smell loss a precise diagnosis whenever this is possible. Any nasal condition which alters the anatomical state of the nose and prevents odours from reaching the olfactory epithelium will impair the sense of smell. The commonest cause of short-term smell loss is the common cold and the most frequent cause of chronic smell loss is rhinitis. Other nasal causes are set out in Table 1.

TESTING THE SENSE OF SMELL

Smell testing involves the preparation and delivery of an odour stimulus and assessment of the response of the olfactory system. This assessment may either be by some form of *objective* measurement of the physiological events produced by the process of olfaction, or it may be by recording the patient's *subjective* response. Objective measurements are unreliable. Recording of olfacto-pupillary and olfacto-respiratory reflexes, and measurement of cardiovascular changes in response to an odour stimulus, have been used in the past. Research is still going on to determine the role of olfactory evoked cortical potentials, analogous to visual evoked responses, but there are many practical difficulties to be overcome. Investigation of the individual's subjective response to the odour stimulus is much more widely used, both clinically and in the context of research, and this approach will accordingly be discussed in more detail.

The simplest form of olfactory testing, and that with which most of us are familiar, is the use of "smell bottles". As carried out in most clinical settings, a set of four or six ageing bottles are found in the back of a cupboard, hastily dusted, and the patient asked to name the odours in the bottles. Even if used properly, there are many disadvantages to this approach. The task of actually *naming* odours, even very familiar ones, presents a challenge quite independent of any impairment of smell itself. Sumner used four well-known smells and investigated 200 subjects without olfactory complaints. He found that only two-thirds of his subjects could name three or more of the four bottles correctly. In many individuals, no more information is gained by using smell bottles than simply by asking them if they have noticed any disturbance of their sense of smell. Performance may be improved, and with it the accuracy of the assessment of olfactory impairment, by eliminating the "free recall" component from the test. This is most easily done by using a "multiple choice" procedure; the patient is given a number of alternative identifications for each smell bottle, and chooses the one which he or she thinks is correct.

Conventional smell bottles are one form of "suprathreshold" test— that is, they are investigating olfactory performance at odour concentrations well above the threshold concentration at which it can be detected and recognised by normal individuals. Another approach to olfactory testing is to measure these threshold concentrations. The *detection threshold* is the lowest concentration of an odour that can be detected as being present. At a higher concentration for each odour is the *recognition threshold,* the minimum concentration for recognition of the odour. Determination of olfactory thresholds in this way is a *quantitative* smell test, as opposed to the *qualitative* test represented by conventional smell bottles. Over the past 100 years or so, many attempts have been made to develop reliable quantitative tests, with varying degrees of success.

Any technique used in quantitative testing is, technically, olfactometry. The use of the word "olfactometer" is, however, usually confined to a piece of equipment designed to prepare and deliver varying concentrations of an olfactory stimulus. Odorants are usually obtained in liquid or solid form and these must be transformed into vapours. Then to obtain the desired concentration of the odorants in air, they can either be diluted with liquid non-smelling solvents or be vaporised and the vapour subsequently diluted with air. A 10-fold concentration increase of the odour may produce only a two-fold or three-fold odour intensity change, as judged by the subject, so the olfactometer must be able to change the concentration of the stimulus over several orders of magnitude if a broad range of responses to any one smell is to be studied.

The most accurate olfactometers in use today use the air dilution principle. The principle is illustrated in Fig. 2, and the model in use at the Smell and Taste Research Center, University of Philadelphia, USA, is shown in Fig. 3. A warmed, filtered and humidified air stream is split into two. One of these streams is then passed through an odorant saturator. The saturated stream is then diluted in various proportions with the unsaturated stream. This produces highly accurate and known concentrations of the odour. This type of olfactometer is too expensive, complex and time consuming for routine use and alternatives more appropriate for the clinical setting must be sought.

Olfactory threshold determinations are most conveniently carried out using a "squeeze bottle" technique (Fig. 4). A number of similar tests are commercially available using different odorants. The test consists of a series of paired bottles. One bottle of the pair contains a known dilution of odorant and the other contains only diluent and acts as a control. The subject is asked to say which of the pair of bottles contains an odour, but is not asked to name the smell. The

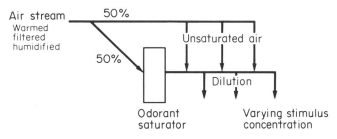

Figure 2: The principle of the air dilution olfactometer.

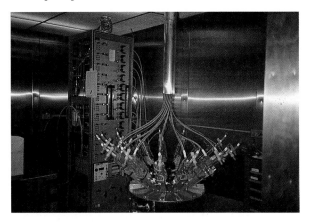

Figure 3: Air dilution olfactometer at the Smell and Taste Research Center, University of Pennsylvania, USA.

weakest concentrations are presented first and a correct choice between odour containing bottle and control bottle has to be made on three separate presentations for that concentration to be taken as the *minimum detectable odour*, or detection threshold. With an experienced tester, the threshold is quickly measured and can be compared with reference values determined empirically from population studies in order to place the test subject into the normal, hyposmic or hyperosmic range.

Threshold evaluation may not, in some patients, correlate closely with impairment of olfactory performance in everyday life. They may have problems with recognition of odours, and this problem is more marked with some odours than others. Suprathreshold measurements obviously have a place, but in view of the drawbacks of conventional smell identification bottles discussed above, consideration must be given to alternative approaches.

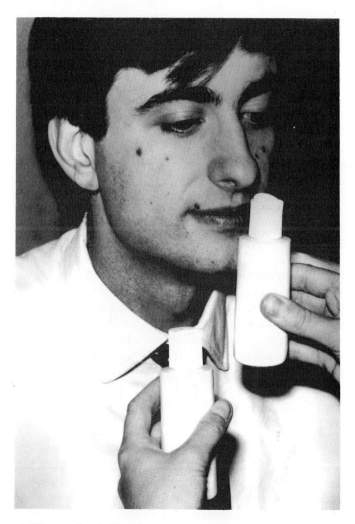

Figure 4: Olfactory threshold testing using PM-carbinol delivered by squeeze bottle. (Olfacto-Labs, 1414 Fourth Street, Berkeley, CA 94710, USA.)

A particularly compact and easy test has been produced by Doty and his colleagues at the University of Pennsylvania, USA. The test is marketed under the title of UPSIT, an acronym for University of Pennsylvania Smell Identification Test. The test comprises 4 booklets containing 10 smells each (Fig. 5). Each of the 10 pages in a book has a strip-shaped area on which the smells are microencapsulated in 10–50 μm crystals. When this odour-impregnated area is scratched with a pencil or fingernail, the smell is released and can be smelt by the subject. This is known colloquially as the "scratch and sniff" technique. On each page are offered four alternative identifications for the smell, and the subject *must* choose one of these identifications, even if apparently nothing can be smelt (i.e. a forced choice technique). Some of the alternatives offered are perhaps inappropriate for the European patient (dill pickle, root beer, pumpkin pie and skunk!) but in general few problems are encountered. Population studies show normal subjects to give 32–40 correct answers, partial anosmics 20–30, and total anosmics—by chance alone—score 7–14 correct answers.

INVESTIGATION OF OLFACTORY DISORDERS

The underlying cause of an olfactory complaint will often be revealed by a detailed history. Particular attention must be paid during the physical examination to the internal anatomy of the nose. A thorough neurological examination will indicate whether the olfactory loss is an isolated problem or part of a more generalised disorder. Depending upon the history and examination, radiography and tomography of the paranasal sinuses and cribriform plate may be indicated.

Olfactory testing should include both threshold and suprathreshold measurements. For threshold measurements a commercially available squeeze-bottle set is appropriate. Suprathreshold testing may be carried out with a set of *at least* eight conventional smell bottles, including a trigeminal stimulant, but more accurate information will be obtained using the UPSIT technique. More complex investigations are rarely used except for research purposes.

TREATMENT OF OLFACTORY DISORDERS

Chronic rhinosinusitis accounts for 30% of cases of smell loss. In this group of patients there is some hope of restoring the sense of smell. The structural changes preventing odours from reaching the olfactory epithelium may not be gross. Minimal oedema around the middle turbinate and upper septum may result in loss of smell even though nasal flow in the rest of the nose is adequate. If simple clinical

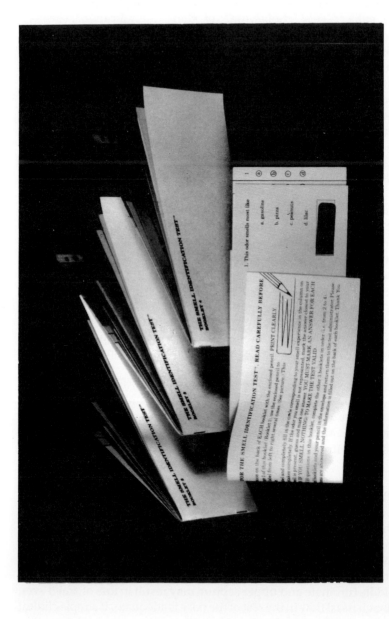

Figure 5: UPSIT—the University of Pennsylvania Smell Identification Test. (Sensonics, 155 Haddon Street, Philadelphia, USA.)

assessment is not adequate, computerised tomography may be of great value.

These patients will have severe hyposmia rather than complete anosmia. Careful smell testing will usually differentiate the two conditions, but in a few individuals the obstruction is so severe that they are indistinguishable. Treatment with topical nasal steroids, or even systemic steroids, may improve airflow sufficiently to establish the correct diagnosis and thereby indicate the possibility that surgical intervention to improve airflow may be helpful. Although these problems of odorant access make up a significant number of cases, useful treatment is not available for many cases of permanent smell loss. In the cases where smell loss can be clearly attributed to zinc and vitamin deficiency, appropriate supplements may improve olfactory function. There is *no* good evidence that they are of any value in other patients with olfactory dysfunction.

CONCLUSION

Smell is evolutionarily the oldest sense. For most of us it is the most evocative sense, the best at stirring old memories, as well as something we use every day. All too often it is ignored by the doctor, but to patients with rhinitis, olfactory disturbance is important—often at least as important as the sensation of nasal obstruction—and these two symptoms deserve equal attention, assessment and treatment.

BIBLIOGRAPHY

Doty RL. A review of olfactory dysfunction in man. *Am J Otolaryngol* 1979; 1: 57–78.
Doty RL, Snow JB. Olfaction. In: Goldman J L, ed. *The principles and practice of rhinology.* Chichester: Wiley Medical. 1987: 761–85.
Meiselman ML, Rivlin RS, eds. *Clinical measurement of taste and smell.* London: Macmillan, 1985.
Moore-Gillon VL. Leading article: testing the sense of smell. *Br Med J* 1987; **294**: 703–4.
Sumner D. On testing the sense of smell. *Lancet* 1962; **ii**: 895–7.

Chapter 6

RADIOLOGY, ULTRASOUND AND ENDOSCOPY IN THE DIAGNOSIS OF DISEASES OF THE NOSE AND PARANASAL SINUSES

W. Draf and G. Strasding

At one time the methods for diagnosis of diseases of the paranasal sinuses were limited to history taking, clinical examination, diaphanoscopy and conventional X-ray. During recent years diagnostic measures have improved significantly.

Sophisticated, but expensive, techniques such as computerised tomography and magnetic resonance imaging allow a detailed examination of the paranasal sinuses. Ultrasound also plays an important role in diagnosis of this type of disease. Finally endoscopy and endoscopic treatment of the nose and its sinuses has been performed for more than 10 years.

This chapter will first explain and compare clinically efficient methods of diagnosis and finally suggest an approach which will enable the general physician to diagnose diseases of the paranasal sinuses and to select the appropriate therapy in cooperation with the specialist.

Before any imaging or invasive diagnostic measures are undertaken, the medical history should be taken and the patient clinically examined. This is the basis for further diagnostics. Radiological, ultrasound and endoscopic findings cannot be interpreted without it.

The otorhinolaryngologist has to use the classical anterior and indirect posterior rhinoscopy. In addition, a microscope and a small flexible endoscope are extremely efficient for examination of the nose and the different ostia of the paranasal sinuses. It is possible to investigate the naso-, oro-, hypopharynx, larynx, and upper trachea as well as the entry to the oesophagus in one examination, in most cases without anaesthesia. Further diagnostic measures depend on the results of these first clinical examinations.

ULTRASOUND

The newest non-invasive imaging method is ultrasound, which has been used in the diagnosis of paranasal sinus diseases since the middle of the 1970s. It is relatively inexpensive and presents no problems to the patient.

A- and B-Scan represent the different ultrasound techniques. The A-Scan (Amplitude modulation) is a one-dimensional method. Like an echosounder, a probe which is put on the tissue's surface sends impulses in short sequences in the ultra-sound range (3.5–5 MegaHz) and receives them again after they have been deflected from tissue borders, like bone, air, soft tissue or liquid. These so-called "echoes" are electronically assimilated and can be seen as an echo-peak on the monitor. The localisation of the peak on the monitor correlates with the geometric distance of the reflecting border area from the ultrasound probe. The height of the peak is related to the intensity of the echo.

In the brightness modulation or B-Scan the sound ray explores the area under investigation in one plane. The reflected echoes are transformed into a scale of grey tones with different degrees of brightness and are shown on the monitor as a two-dimensional sectional view with correct reproduction of areas and angles.

Both techniques can be applied to the examination of the paranasal sinuses, but the A-Scan is used more frequently whereas the B-Scan is used to explore the soft tissue of the neck, and the salivary glands.

In order to interpret the findings it is necessary to understand the properties of sound, especially of ultrasound. Because ultrasound can spread better in a solid or liquid medium than in air, it is more difficult to examine, for example, the air-containing maxillary sinus than soft tissue and vessels of the neck, which consist of solid and liquid media. Fig. 1 shows an example of an A-Scan picture in which only the initial echo can be seen on the monitor. This echo has to be assigned to the structure which is located closest to the probe, in this case the anterior wall of the maxillary sinus. Further deflections of the cathode ray cannot be seen. Therefore, one has to suppose an air-containing maxillary sinus. In the gaseous medium the sound cannot spread enough and is barely reflected from the next bordering area, the posterior wall of the maxillary sinus. One has to bear in mind that all pathological findings cannot be seen in an ultrasound examination of the paranasal sinuses if there is air in front of them. The isolated

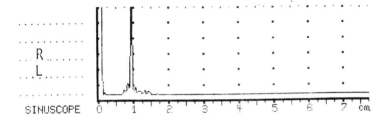

Figure 1: A-scan of the maxillary sinus with no pathological findings

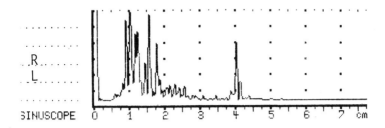

Figure 2: A-scan of the maxillary sinus with mucosal swelling and secretion

maxillary sinus polyp or the isolated cyst of the posterior maxillary sinus wall is not seen in this instance.

The example in Fig. 2 shows a maxillary sinus with mucosal swelling, filled with secretory product. Here the sound can spread easily; it is reflected from the posterior wall of the maxillary sinus and can be seen as a final echo-peak on the monitor according to the depth of the maxillary sinus. The echoes following the initial peak represent the mucosal swelling.

Allowing for the possibility of air concealing nasal pathology, mucosal swellings, polyps, cysts and various secretory products such as pus and blood can be differentiated by ultrasound examination.

The same physical constraints apply to the B-scan. The air-conditioning maxillary sinus is free of echo, but if the maxillary sinus is filled with secretion, the posterior wall of the maxillary sinus can be seen on the monitor as a horizontal or vertical sectional view, depending on the position of the probe (Fig. 3.a,b).

Ultrasound imaging of the paranasal sinuses is therefore useful for viewing the maxillary and frontal sinuses. For the ethmoidal cell system it is not of great value and the sphenoid sinus cannot be examined by this method.

83

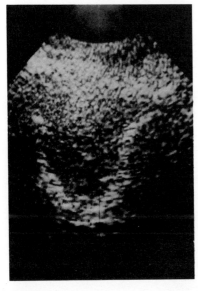

Figure 3a(Left): B-scan of the maxillary sinus containing secretion and polypous mucosal swelling

Figure 3b: Explanatory diagram for 3a

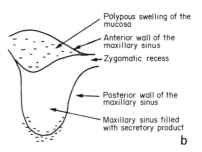

Polypous swelling of the mucosa

Anterior wall of the maxillary sinus

Zygomatic recess

Posterior wall of the maxillary sinus

Maxillary sinus filled with secretory product

b

X-ray[1]

X-ray examination of the paranasal sinuses is a test of proven value which has been in use for a long time. Nowadays computer tomography and occasionally magnetic resonance imaging can be used in addition to conventional X-ray techniques. The plain radiograph of the maxillary sinus in the occipito-dental ray-path, known as Water's view, is the most important X-ray technique. This method allows the maxillary sinuses to be seen free of parts of the petrous bone. The frontal sinuses are enlarged and clearly visible, and the sphenoid sinuses are projected into the open mouth. The ethmoid sinuses cannot be seen so well, because the nasal bones cover parts of the ethmoid cells (Fig. 4).

If a demonstration of the ethmoid sinuses is specifically required, the occipito-frontal variation of Water's view is more suitable. With this technique the frontal sinuses are shown in their natural size. Normally both X-ray techniques are combined, and completed by an X-ray of the frontal sinuses from the lateral view (Fig. 5.a,b).

An occipito-nasal X-ray of the paranasal sinus system can reveal involvement of the orbit in its processes due to tumour growth or fractures of the paranasal sinuses, especially the floor of the orbit

[1]We appreciate the support of Prof. Dr. J.-P. Haas, Head of the Institute for Radiology, Fulda (X-rays, CT-Scans etc.)

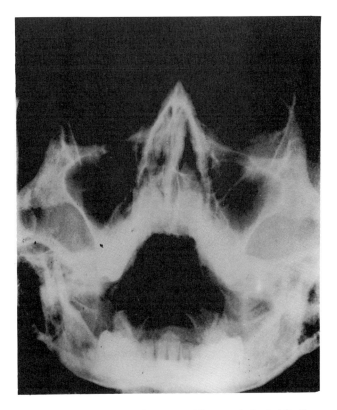

Figure 4: Water's view of paranasal sinuses without pathological findings

(Fig. 6), while an axial X-ray of the skull base shows the sphenoid sinus and ethmoidal cell system from below (Fig. 7).

All of these techniques can be usefully employed in screening for cases of inflammatory and tumorous conditions of the paranasal sinus system and fractures of the midface. Liquid accumulations can be differentiated from soft tissue processes by the typical fluid level, which can be demonstrated by various tilt views. Soft tissue processes are represented by opacity of diverse density and form.

More precise information about the extent of the pathological findings seen in the simple X-ray can be gathered with conventional sagittal and, if necessary, lateral computer tomography (CT) of the paranasal sinus system. With this technique the area to be examined is demonstrated in cross sections of approximately 5 mm from posterior to anterior with a small amount of overlapping. In this way one can obtain information about the location of osseous defects in

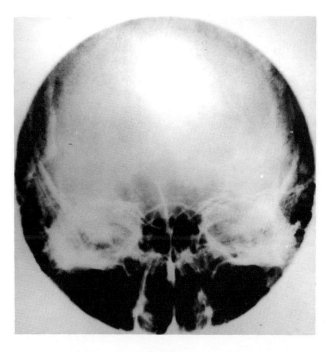

Figure 5a: Occipito-frontal variation of Water's view. Paranasal sinuses without pathological findings

the case of tumours or fractures of the paranasal sinuses. However, conventional tomography has become less important for diagnosis in the head and neck region since the development of high-resolution-computer tomography.

High resolution CT is performed in an axial and coronal projection. The smallest possible cross section is 1 mm and the thickness of the individual cuts can be chosen by computer program, depending on the problem. In this way it is possible to get a very detailed image of the paranasal sinus system.

Computerised multiplanar reconstructions in various projections (axial, coronal, sagittal) allow the exact allocation of pathological findings to the anatomical structures of the paranasal sinuses. The surgeon gets a three-dimensional image of the process (Figs. 8a–c).

The indications for computer tomography are similar to those for the conventional techniques—the detailed exploration of inflammatory or tumorous processes, malformations or fractures in the whole system, including ethmoidal cells and the sphenoid

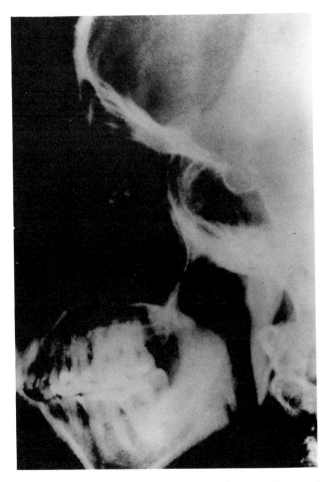

Figure 5b. Lateral projection showing a plain frontal sinus without pathological findings

sinus. The surgeon is provided with a good view over neighbouring structures such as the optic nerve and the canals of the carotid arteries. Preoperative surgical planning is made easier, because tissue, bones and air can be clearly distinguished. Inside the soft tissue there are further possibilities for differentiation by measurement of the density of liquid accumulation.

Magnetic resonance imaging (MRI) which is still very expensive, is always indicated when an endocranial complication is suspected. It can also be useful when it is difficult to differentiate between an

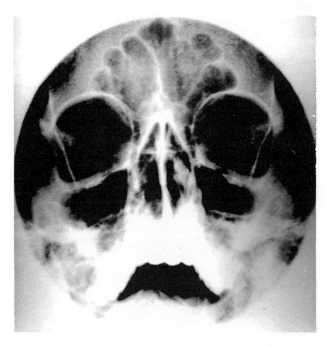

Figure 6: Occipito-nasal projection of paranasal sinuses with no pathological findings

inflammatory and tumorous disease of the nose and paranasal sinus system with computer tomography. The major disadvantage of MRI is the inability to demonstrate osseous structures.

ENDOSCOPY OF THE NOSE AND PARANASAL SINUSES

Endoscopic techniques became popular in hospitals and general practice following the development of thin telescopes (2.7–4 mm in diameter) with high light intensity by Hopkins. Since it is possible to examine the frontal, sphenoid and maxillary sinuses endoscopically, it seems more logical to use the terms ''endoscopy of the maxillary, frontal or sphenoid sinus'' and ''endoscopy of paranasal sinuses'' rather than ''sinuscopy'', ''sinoscopy'' or ''Highmoroscopy'' which were used formerly. Both rigid and flexible endoscopes are available.

Endoscopy of the nose and paranasal sinuses is generally performed as an outpatient procedure with the patient recumbent and locally anaesthetised. In adults this type of surgery is done

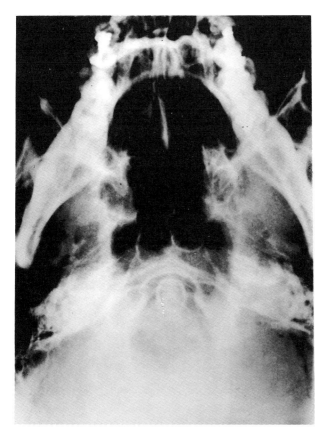

Figure 7. Axial X-ray of the skull base, showing sphenoid sinus and ethmoidal cell system with no pathological findings

under general anaesthesia if further endoscopies are planned for the same session. In nasal endoscopy one examines from posterior to anterior the lower, middle and inferior nasal meatus. We prefer the canine fossa as the approach to the maxillary sinus, because it allows better mobility of the instruments for inspection of the ostium and for the surgical procedures (Fig. 9).

In children under eight or nine years endoscopy is performed by way of the inferior nasal meatus in order not to endanger the tooth buds of final dentition. We also use the inferior nasal meatus as an approach if it is likely that fenestration of the maxillary sinus will follow.

During endoscopy it is possible to remove solitary cysts and

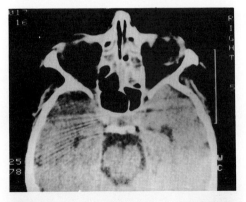

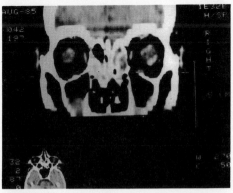

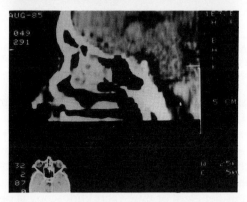

Figure 8a – c: Computerised multiplanar reconstructions of a parallel sinus system with opacity of the ethmoidal cell system and partial opacity of the maxillary sinuses. Frontal and sphenoid sinuses with no pathological findings.
8a Axial projection
8b Coronal reconstruction
8c Sagittal reconstruction

90

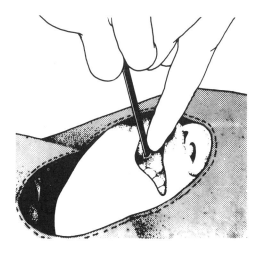

Figure 9: Endoscopy of the right maxillary sinus via the canine fossa

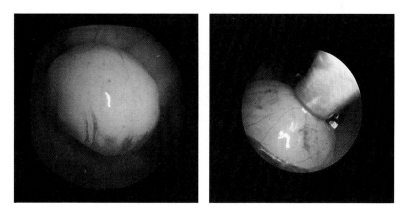

Figure 10a: (Left) Solitary cyst in the maxillary sinus
Figure 10b: (Right) Extraction of the cyst by optical biopsy forceps

polyps in the maxillary sinus under optical control (Figs. 10a,b) and also to take biopsies. Besides assessing the integrity of the mucous membrane of the paranasal sinuses it is also possible to reveal tissue eosinophilia in cases of allergic disease.

In contrast to endoscopy of the maxillary sinus, endoscopy of the frontal sinus is seldom indicated, but it can also prove of value. In this technique a 6 mm wide hole is drilled into the anterior wall of the frontal sinus after a small skin incision is made at the medial end of the eyebrow. The trocar and telescope can then be inserted.

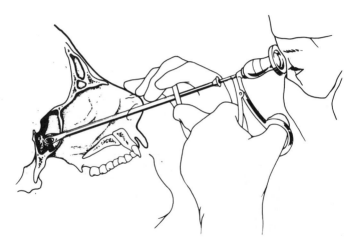

Figure 11: Endoscopy of the sphenoid sinus with an extra-long trocar; biopsy

Depending on the finding, local therapy or a larger intervention may follow. Endoscopy of the sphenoid sinus is indicated for particular diagnostic purposes: 1. Unclear radiological findings; 2. If a tumour is suspected and if there is no other way of obtaining a biopsy (e.g. from the nasopharynx); 3. To diagnose a CSF-fistula in frontobasal fractures; 4. Intraoperatively in fractures of the sphenoid sinus and control after hypophysectomy. The sphenoid sinus is opened transnasally close to the midline and the floor with an extra-long trocar (Fig. 11).

General indications for endoscopy of the paranasal sinuses are negative X-ray findings in cases of clinically suspicious symptoms like recurrent nose bleed, blocked nose, indefinite pain, search for primary tumour and the diagnosis of liquor fistula. An unclear radiographic finding with or without minor symptoms is also an indication for endoscopy as well as negative irrigation results, radiographically demonstrated swelling of the mucosa, search for a "focus", previous operation of an antrum and exclusion of a neoplasm. Endoscopic inspection of the paranasal sinuses helps to determine whether diseases of the surrounding area have involved the paranasal sinuses.

Finally observation to assess the effects of treatment in malignant diseases is safer with endoscopy. Figures 12–14 show a few typical examples.

Side effects and complications after endoscopy of the nose and paranasal sinuses are rare. Temporary paraesthesia sometimes

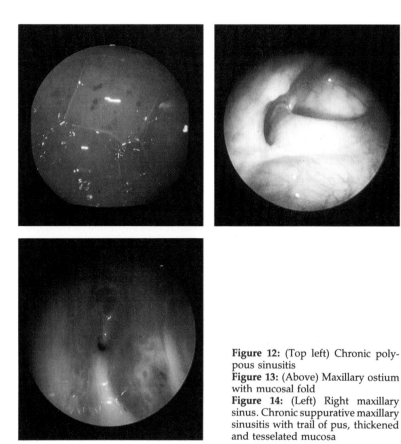

Figure 12: (Top left) Chronic poly-pous sinusitis
Figure 13: (Above) Maxillary ostium with mucosal fold
Figure 14: (Left) Right maxillary sinus. Chronic suppurative maxillary sinusitis with trail of pus, thickened and tesselated mucosa

occurs in the region of the incisor and canine teeth after endoscopy of the maxillary sinus. For two days the patient should refrain from nose blowing, otherwise a minor skin emphysema may occur. Severe complications and injuries of the neighbouring structures, or the frightening air-embolism which can occur after blind irrigation, have not been seen with endoscopy.

During endoscopy of the frontal sinus the supraorbital nervé has to be preserved, in order to avoid paresthesia or hypaesthesia in the region innervated by it. If the sphenoid sinus is inspected, one must be very careful in order to avoid damaging the neighbouring internal carotid artery or causing a liquor fistula. If there is a spontaneous

93

dehiscence of the bone to the optic nerve canal, or if the bony canal is destroyed by a tumour, loss of sight may occur, but this is extremely rare.

VALUE OF THE DIFFERENT EXAMINATION METHODS
(FIG. 15)

Each clinical assessment starts with history taking and physical examination. Pathological changes in the nose, its turbinates, the nasal meatus and the paranasal sinus ostia may become apparent during anterior and posterior rhinoscopy and rigid and flexible endoscopy.

In experienced hands ultrasound can reveal significant changes in the maxillary and frontal sinus such as secretion, swelling of the mucosa, and even cysts and polyps. Neither conservative nor surgical treatment should be initiated solely on the results of ultrasound investigations. For follow-up after therapy, however, ultrasound examination is sufficient in many cases. This avoids unnecessary numbers of X-rays and reduces the exposure to radiation which is especially important in pregnant women and children.

If, following clinical and ultrasound examination a disease of the paranasal sinuses is not suspected, an X-ray is not necessary. However, if a disease is suspected, further radiological or/and endoscopic measures are necessary to achieve a clear diagnosis *before* a specific therapy is begun. Negative ultrasound findings, persistent complaints, resistance to therapy and unclear ultrasound results demand further radiological interventions. ''Water's view'' X-ray can be valuable in these circumstances.

Computer tomography is indicated in cases of severe complaints and relatively discrete clinical and radiological findings in a Water's view X-ray, and also if several sinuses are involved. Before any major surgical intervention of the paranasal sinuses, high resolution computer tomography should be performed. Post-operative follow-up by CT also provides more precise information than was previously available.

High resolution CT is preferable to conventional CT, because only in this way can the very thin osseous structures such as those of the ethmoidal cell system be seen, even in cases of severe polyposis. CT is the imaging method of choice if malformations are expected, and in injuries of the facial skeleton.

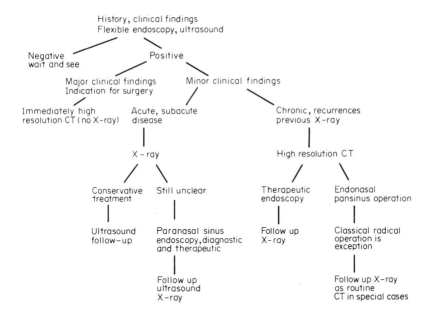

Figure 15: Diagnostics and therapy in inflammatory diseases of the nose and paranasal sinuses

For simultaneous identification and therapy of radiologically discovered localised alterations of the paranasal sinus system, or for taking biopsies, paranasal sinus endoscopy is the diagnostic method of choice. Examination of the maxillary, frontal and sphenoid sinus, including biopsy, is also possible independent of the radiological findings. If the aim is to achieve a clear paranasal sinus diagnosis and possibly to perform subsequent endoscopic therapy, (as, for example, in chronic purulent sinusitis) endoscopy is indicated as a less traumatising method.

The classical puncture and blind irrigation of the maxillary sinus, which is painful to the patient, gives a relatively clear result only if the irrigation and aspiration findings are positive. Therefore this method is almost obsolete nowadays, except for a few special cases.

Endoscopic therapy closes a gap between the extremes of conservative therapy on the one hand and radical paranasal sinus surgery on the other. To the benefit of patients, the number of radical paranasal sinus operations can be reduced and the success rate of such interventions increased because of a more precise indication.

In conclusion ultrasound and X-ray examination can be used individually or together for the diagnosis of paranasal sinus diseases, following detailed clinical examination. High resolution computer tomography is a further aid to diagnosis, which plays an important role before major surgical therapy.

Investigation of suspicious clinical and radiographic findings can be combined with possible therapy in endoscopy of paranasal sinuses (Fig. 15). This is especially important because the findings of conventional X-ray examination and the findings in maxillary sinus endoscopy can differ to a remarkable extent.

BIBLIOGRAPHY

Brusis T, Mödder U. *HNO-Röntgen-Aufnahmetechnik und Normalbefunde*. Heidelberg, New York, Tokyo: Springer, 1984.

Draf W. *Endoscopy of the paranasal sinuses*. Heidelberg, New York, Tokyo: Springer, 1983.

Draf W. Endoskopie der Nase und der Nasennebenhöhlen. *Dt Ärzteblatt* 1983; **9**: 25–32.

Mann WJ. *Ultraschall im Kopf-Hals-Bereich*. Heidelberg, New York, Tokyo: Springer, 1984.

Chapter 7

SEASONAL RHINITIS

R. Davies

HISTORICAL BACKGROUND

Rather suprisingly, seasonal allergic rhinitis is a disease of modern times, hardly recognised in antiquity. Although rare descriptions can be identified in Islamic texts from the 9th century and European writings of the 16th century, seasonal rhinitis was adequately described only in the early 19th century, and at that time it was regarded as a most unusual condition. Up until the 17th century nasal catarrh was thought to be a secretion from the brain and the earliest association of seasonal rhinitis was with roses, hence its initial classification as "the rose cold".

The London physician, John Bostock, collected some cases together calling the condition summer catarrh or *catarrhus aestivus,* but remarked that the disease had hardly been noticed until the previous ten years. His researches indicated that summer catarrh only occurred "In the middle or upper classes of Society, some indeed of high rank. I made enquiry at the various dispensaries in London and elsewhere but I have not heard of a single unequivocal case occurring amongst the poor". Bostock thought that hay fever was caused by heated air, sunshine or the use of bodily exercise.

Charles Blackley, who was himself a hay fever sufferer, published his book *Experimental researches on the cause and nature of catarrhus aestivus* in 1893 (Fig. 1). In this book he unequivocally identified pollens from grass as the cause of hay fever. He was the first to perform the critical experiments showing that pollen put into the nose reproduced symptoms of hay fever, and put into the eyes produced conjunctivitis. He was one of the first to perform allergy skin testing and also showed the height at which pollen grains travelled in the atmosphere by attaching sticky plates to kites. It was at about this time that the incidence of hay fever began to increase and Blackley made the interesting observation that "the persons

EXPERIMENTAL RESEARCHES

ON THE

CAUSES AND NATURE

OF

CATARRHUS AESTIVUS

(HAY-FEVER OR HAY-ASTHMA)

BY

CHARLES H. BLACKLEY, M.R.C.S. ENG.

*'When a small portion of pollen, just enough to tinge
the tip of the finger yellow, was applied to the mucous
membrane of the nares, some of the symptoms of hay
fever were invariably developed, the severity and
continuance of which were dependent on the quality
and on the number of times it was used.'*

LONDON:
BAILLIÈRE, TINDALL & COX,
KING WILLIAM STREET, STRAND.

PARIS: BAILLIÈRE | MADRID: BAILLIÈRE.

1873.

Figure 1: Frontispiece of Charles Blackley's book.

who are most subjected to the action of pollen belong to a class which
furnishes the fewest cases of the disorder, namely the farming
classes. This remarkable fact may be accounted for in two different
ways. It may on the one hand be due to the absence of the
predisposition which mental culture generates, or on the other hand
it may be in this disease there is a possibility of a patient being
rendered insusceptible to the action of pollen by continued exposure
to its influence''. He underlined the traditional view that hay fever
was a disease predominantly of the upper cultured classes, and
introduced the idea that individuals could be rendered insusceptible
to the effects of pollen, leading the way for the desensitisation
injection therapy introduced by Noon and Freeman, some 40 years
later.

By the early 20th century hay fever was common, so much so that
the *General Practitioner Journal* reviewing the book on *Hay Fever* by
William Lloyd of London began with a comment to the effect that
''From our point of view this book is important, firstly because it
treats a very common complaint''.

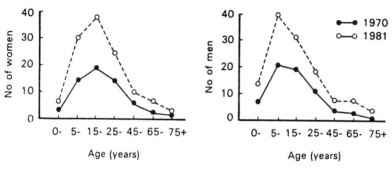

Number of patients consulting their family doctor for treatment for rhinitis in 1970 and 1981

Figure 2: Prevalence of hay fever in general practice (From Fleming DM, Crombie DL. *Br Med J* 1987; **294**: 279–83. Reproduced by kind permission of the Editor, *British Medical Journal*.)

EPIDEMIOLOGY

In 1979 John Fry classed hay fever as one of the commonest diseases of general practice in the United Kingdom. He found that the cumulative incidence of hay fever amongst those seeking medical advice in his practice was 7%, and at least 2% would be expected to present in any one year for medical treatment. This would represent at least one million people attending their family practitioner every year for treatment for hay fever. More recent large scale surveys in general practice have indicated that the prevalence of hay fever, at least as judged by patients attending their family doctors for treatment, has doubled in the last 10 years, and it is likely that this is an under-estimate of the true prevalence of the disease. Patients attending their general practitioners for treatment probably represent less than half of those who suffer since many afflicted by seasonal rhinitis treat themselves. The disease is equally common in both sexes, its incidence being highest between the ages of 15 and 25 (Fig. 2). The overall estimates of approximately 10% of the population suffering from hay fever in the United Kingdom is very similar to that for the United States of America.

Unfortunately there are no comprehensive longitudinal studies on hay fever to prove that the disease has actually increased in frequency, though review of the historical perspective of this disease strongly suggests that it has. As originally pointed out by Blackley, there is the curious phenomenon that hay fever is apparently less common in rural than in urban areas, suggesting that those regularly exposed to grass develop tolerance to pollen allergens. Certainly prior to the industrial revolution the bulk of the population lived on the land and were exposed to pollen even in winter when hay was fed to cattle indoors, and tolerance may have developed to the relatively constant exposure to the lower concentrations of pollen that were found at that time. The increase in grass production and seasonal exposure only of those living in towns may have led to the development of sensitivity to pollen and with it, hay fever. However, over the last 30 years there has been a steady decline in the amount of pollen present in the air in the summer in the United Kingdom. There are many reasons for this, the first being the increased use of silage as cattle fodder. Grass is cut in May for silage before the majority has had time to pollinate. In addition the increased use of Timothy and Rye grasses which are poorer pollen producers than Cocksfoot grass has also contributed to the lower pollen counts. On this basis alternative causes need to be identified for the increasing prevalence of hay fever.

Whilst pollen grains have declined, the amount of air pollutants present in the air has increased six-fold in the last 30 years and it is certainly possible that ozone and the oxides of sulphur and nitrogen could have led to damage to the respiratory tract epithelium, allowing allergens better access to the immune system. Cigarette smoking may well have led to an increase in atopy; certainly there is evidence that children exposed to cigarette smoke in the home are more likely to develop atopic diseases.

AETIOLOGY

Pollen is the major cause of allergic disease throughout the world, the most important being those that rely upon the wind for pollination and of these, grasses are the most important. Consisting of roughly 9000 species, grasses cover 20% of the world's surface. Their flowers open only for a few hours a day to permit pollination and the pollen itself, 20-30μ in diameter, is viable for less than a day. The pollen season is related to the cycle of plant development. In temperate climates grasses begin to flower in May and the peak season for grass pollenosis in the majority of sufferers is June and July. In equatorial regions the seasonal effect is largely absent. Weed pollen allergies vary with the geographical location. In Northern Europe the common stinging nettle produces pollen during the summer and autumn, whereas another member of the same family,

Parietaria judeaica, is the most important pollen allergen in Southern Italy. Recently cases of allergy to Parietaria have been described in Southern England. In North America the pollen that effects most atopic people is that produced in the autumn by a species of ragweed which is largely absent from Europe. Ragweed consists of the common and giant species. They are unsightly plants found on low ground, along the side of streams and in waste places. They represent the most troublesome cause of hay fever in both North America and probably in Japan. Ragweed flowers in late summer and autumn and at peak times there may be over 1000 pollen grains per cubic metre air. Another weed important in allergic rhinitis is *Artemesia vulgaris*, the common mugwort. It is difficult to find a country in Northern Europe in which this weed does not grow, though its importance as a cause of pollinosis appears to be diminishing, largely due to the use of weedkillers. Its pollen is produced during the late summer and autumn. Bermuda grass *Cynodon dactylon* is a creeping, low growing, greyish grass commonly found in lawns in tropical areas since it is one of the few grasses that can survive high temperatures. It is an important cause of pollinosis in the summer months in the United States, South America and throughout the warmer countries of the world. However, in cooler areas, such as the United Kingdom, Timothy grass, Rye grass and Cocksfoot predominate (Fig. 3). Cocksfoot (*Dactylis glomerata*) is an early flowering species shedding its pollen in June, but now only accounts for 2% of grass seed that is planted. Both Timothy grass (*Phleum pratense*) and Rye grass (*Lolium perenne*) are poorer pollen producers and pollinate later in the summer. These changes in sown grasses may account for the gradual reduction in pollen counts that has been seen over the last 30 years. For example between 1961 and 1970 the mean daily pollen count during June and July did not fall below 50, whereas it dropped to 39 during the decade from 1971 to 1980 and is still falling.

It has been shown that the majority of patients with hay fever experience symptoms once the number of grass pollen grains in the air reaches 50 per cubic metre. When there has been a warm spring this concentration of grass pollen in the air occurs as early as the first week of June. However, if the spring is cold then it is unlikely that these pollen counts will be achieved until the last two weeks of June. The pollen concentration on any day during the grass pollen season is determined mainly by the weather. In general rain washes the air clean and high wind speeds lead to low pollen concentrations. There is considerable cross reactivity between the allergens present in the

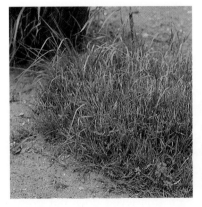 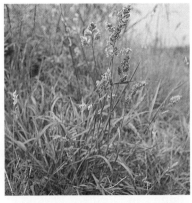

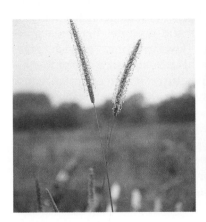 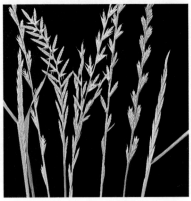

Timothy grass

Rye grass

Figure 3

common grass pollens encountered in the United Kingdom. It is of interest to note that the pollen counts experienced in the United Kingdom do not approach those experienced during the ragweed season in the United States of America.

Whilst pollens from grasses and weeds can cause symptoms from early summer through to the autumn, spring-time allergic rhinitis is the result of allergy to tree pollens (Fig. 4). Probably the most important pollen producers are trees of the birch family. In the United Kingdom the silver birch is an ornamental tree grown in gardens in the suburbs of many cities, but in Northern Europe and North America the tree is of considerable economic importance. The

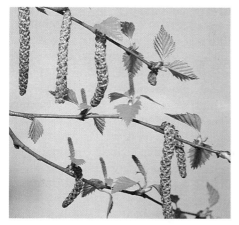

Figure 4:
Left: Male and female catkins of silver birch.
Below left: Japanese red cedar.
Below right: Flowers of the common oak.

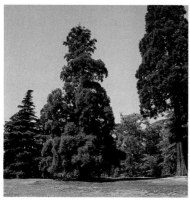

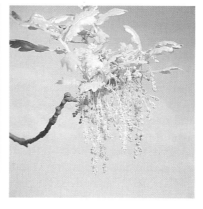

bark and wood of the birch trees is waterproof, a fact recognised by the North American indians who use birch to build canoes and wigwams. Birch trees are also found in the Alps where it is a potent pollen producer causing allergic symptoms in March and April. The first of the pollens encountered as early as February is that from the hazel tree. In fact the pollen develops in the late sumnmer, matures over the winter and is released early in the year causing allergic rhinitis in February and March. Plane trees are particularly common in many cities and pollinate in the early summer. Pollen from oak trees found extensively in the northern hemisphere generally causes symptoms in the late spring and early summer. Some trees and their pollens only cause allergic rhinitis in particular countries. For example, in Japan the cedar or Sugi tree is an evergreen growing 30–50 metres tall and it the most important tree grown for timber. Up to a third of cultivated land in Japan is devoted to growing these trees and allergy to its pollen is extremely common, causing symptoms in March and April. The mesquite is a medium sized deciduous tree armed with spines up to 5cm long, the fruits are pods which in some areas are ground for food. The green, sweet smelling flowers appear early in the summer. Mesquite is widely found in the southern states of America and its recent introduction into the Middle East has caused pollinosis to develop for the first time.

Fungal spores are approximately $5\mu m$ in diameter and are too small to be impacted into the eye to cause allergic conjunctivitis. However, they can cause allergic rhinitis and many cases of summertime and early autumn rhinitis are due to allergy to Cladosporium and Alternaria. Spore counts can be very high, for example in London Cladosporium concentrations reach 10 000 and Alternaria 1000 spores per cubic metre air. They are an important cause of allergy, accounting for up to a fifth of cases of rhinitis during the late summer months. Cladosporium spores are released into the air when lawns are mown, and Alternaria during the harvest time. Damp conditions inside houses lead to the growth of moulds particularly of the genus Penicillium. This mould, as well as Cladosporium, can colonise wallpaper and even painted surfaces, and may account for allergic symptoms in sufferers living in damp dwellings. In temperate climates the spores of *Aspergillus fumigatus* occur in the air throughout the year. The fungus colonises decaying vegetation and is common in mouldy hay. Spores are commonest in the early winter and, though not particularly associated with the development of allergic rhinitis, are the cause of allergic bronchopulmonary aspergillosis, a disease causing asthma and pulmonary eosinophilia.

PATHOPHYSIOLOGY

The irritation, sneezing and hypersecretion that follows exposure to allergen almost certainly results from stimulation of H_1 receptors on sensory nerve endings by histamine. Further increases in nasal secretion and dilatation of glandular vessels which accompany the allergic response are due to reflex activation of parasympathetic nerves which release acetylcholine and vasoactive intestinal polypeptide (VIP). The evidence for the reflex nature of this event comes from studies on the effect of unilateral nasal provocation with histamine or allergen. In either case stimulation of one nostril causes

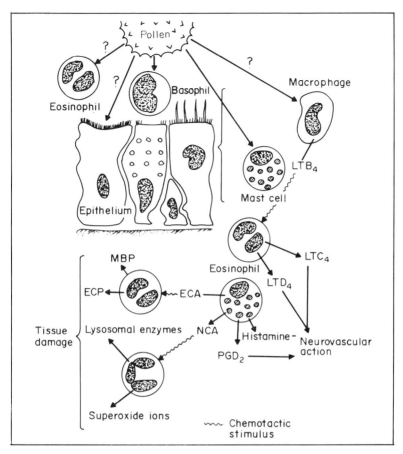

Figure 5: Pathophysiology of rhinitis

a secretory response in both, though the amount secreted from the provoked nostril is greater. However, unilateral provocation does not significantly change the contralateral airway resistance. The increase in nasal resistance in the challenged nostril is thought to be due mainly to the effects of mediators from mast and probably other cells acting directly on blood vessels, causing swelling of the venous erectile tissue. Whilst histamine causes nasal vasodilatation with venocongestion through H_1 and H_2 receptors, the role of other mediators in the nose remains more speculative. However, it is likely that one of the sulphidopeptide leukotrienes, namely leukotriene D4, which on topical administration causes substantial nasal congestion, is likely to be of importance in the pathogenesis of allergic rhinitis (Fig. 5).

The effectiveness of antihistaminic drugs in the management of allergic rhinitis has underlined the importance of the mast cells in this disease. Histological studies have shown that there are more mast cells present in the nasal mucous membrane of atopic rhinitic patients compared to non-atopic non-rhinitic subjects and that the total number of mast cells increases up to eight-fold during the summer months in patients allergic to grass pollen. Further, there is an increase in the proportion of these cells in the surface epithelium at this time, where they are ideally placed to interact with pollen settling on the nasal mucosa. In addition, the experimental instillation of aqueous extract of grass pollen into the nose of sensitised individuals causes a substantial and significant increase in the number of mast cells showing features of degranulation.

The majority of nasal mast cells, like those in the mucosa of the lower respiratory tract, differ from mast cells in human skin or in the submucosa of intestinal tract, in that they do not readily stain with safranine O and do not degranulate on contact with the polyamine 40/80. In addition, fixation with formal saline as opposed to Carnoy's solution reduces the number of mast cells which can be detected following staining with Alcian blue or by the alpha naphthol ASD chloracetate esterase reaction. Such cells in the bronchial epithelium have been shown to contain tryptase as the major neutral protease, whereas mast cells in human skin also contain a second neutral protease, chymotrypsin. The significance of these differences in the characteristics of mast cells in different organs of the body, and indeed in different sites within the same organ, is as yet undetermined. It is possible that there are different types of mast cells which congregate in different parts of the body. Alternatively the characteristics of mast cells may differ in response to the local environment being influenced by adjacent cells.

Nasal lavage has consistently shown increases in both histamine and the mast cell derived prostenoid prostaglandin D2 (PDG_2) following introduction of ragweed pollen grains into the nose, confirming the importance of mast cell degranulation in the immediate nasal response to allergen. In contrast to the lower respiratory tract, late phase reactions in the nose are more difficult to detect and occur at different times in different patients. Nasal lavage during such reactions has shown the presence of histamine, leukotriene C4 (LTC_4) and albumin, but not prostaglandin D2 suggesting involvement of basophils in which PGD_2 is not a major cyclooxygenase product rather than mast cells. Whether or not basophils really are important in the late phase reaction in the human nose remains to be determined. It is probable that the events that occur during the late nasal response to allergen are important in the ongoing symptoms of seasonal rhinitis, yet the mechanisms causing persistent nasal blockage in this condition remain unknown. Stimulation of nasal sensory nerve endings by histamine is known to produce irritation, sneezing, discharge and an increase in nasal airways resistance. In allergic rhinitis however, antihistamines have only a minimal effect on nasal blockage indicating that vasodilators other than histamine are involved in the pathophysiology of this condition. Substance P and VIP are present in nasal mucosal sensory and parasympathetic nerve fibres respectively. Although these mediators and PGE_2 are known to produce vasodilatation of nasal resistance vessels there is no direct evidence of their involvement in allergic rhinitis. Furthermore PGE_2 acts as a vasoconstrictor of capacitance vessels.

It is, however, possible that the sulphidopeptide leukotrienes, particularly LTD_4, which are found in secretions and are known to be released from eosinophils could play an important role in persistent nasal congestion. There is accumulating evidence to support an important role for the eosinophil in the development of allergic rhinitis. Seasonal increases in numbers of eosinophils, neutrophils and lymphocytes can be shown in nasal lavage in patients with allergic rhinitis due to grass pollen and a close correlation has been found between the number of eosinophils in nasal or epithelial tissue and nasal symptoms and the pollen counts. Further, biopsies have shown an increased number of eosinophils in the nasal mucous membrane during the grass pollen season compared with out of the season in patients with hay fever.

Studies on the histological changes in nasal tissue at intervals during the 24 hours following instillation of allergen into one nostril have shown that mast cell numbers decreased within one hour not only in the nostril challenged with allergen but also in the unchallenged nostril, indicating the possibility that mast cell degranulation can occur in response to a nasal reflex. However, the importance of the eosinophil in the subsequent nasal response is indicated by the fact that there is a transient but significant increase in eosinophil numbers only in the challenge nostril. The transient nature of the tissue infiltration with eosinophils is probably related to the fact that these cells move through the mucosa into the secretions. The fact that eosinophil accumulation occurs only in the nostril challenged with allergen, suggests chemoattraction is by mechanisms that do not include mast cells, perhaps by release of chemoattractants such as LTB$_4$ from macrophages or interleukin-5 from T lymphocytes of which there are a great many in the cell-rich subepithelial layer of the human nasal mucosa.

Although eosinophils can liberate platelet activating factor (PAF) the role of this mediator in nasal allergic reactions remains uncertain, since topical application leads to vasoconstriction of capacitance vessels within the nasal mucosa reducing nasal airway resistance. Further, activation of eosinophils is associated with the release of proteins cytotoxic for respiratory epithelium, such as major basic (MBP) and cationic proteins (ECP). However, there is no evidence of loss of the nasal epithelium in the course of seasonal allergic rhinitis.

DIAGNOSIS

The diagnosis of seasonal rhinitis is straightforward. Its common incidence means that everyone knows somebody among their family or friends who suffers from this condition and with whom symptoms can be compared. The critical factor in the diagnosis is the seasonality of the symptoms occurring in the UK between April and September. It is rare to develop infectious rhinitis during this period of time and this condition can usually be distinguished from allergic rhinitis by the presence of pharyngeal pain, thicker yellow-green nasal discharge and more generalised symptoms including malaise. In allergic rhinitis nasal secretions are usually thin and watery, and symptoms vary on a day-to-day basis according to exposure to allergens. In addition the time course of allergic rhinitis is subsequently longer than that of the infectious disease.

Seasonal rhinitis is rarely associated with the problems that are common in the perennial form of the disease where, for example, sinusitis is common. In children the allergic salute (rubbing of the nose to separate the swollen nasal mucosal surfaces) and a horizontal bar or crease on the nose caused by continual rubbing may be seen. Of course patients with seasonal rhinitis may in addition suffer from perennial rhinitis in which case more troublesome and persistent signs and symptoms of the disease will be present.

IDENTIFICATION OF THE ALLERGIC CAUSE

A recent survey indicated the months at which patients suffering from allergic rhinitis considered that their symptoms were at their

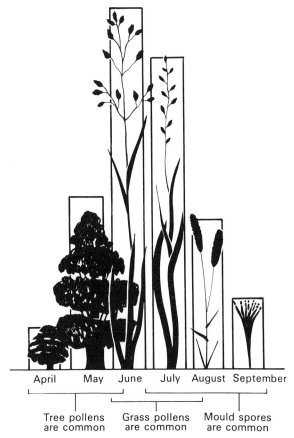

Figure 6: Maximum symptoms of hay fever and allergens

worst. This is illustrated in Fig. 6 in relation to the main allergic causes of seasonal rhinitis. It is clear that June remains the month during which the majority of patients suffering from allergic rhinitis are at their worst. Clearly individuals whose seasonal rhinitis is mainly due to allergy to tree pollens are worst in April and May whilst grass typically causes symptoms from May through to August. The autumn is characterised by allergic rhinitis due to the presence of moulds.

INVESTIGATION

The investigation of seasonal rhinitis requires no more than a careful history. Skin testing is unlikely to reveal any additional information that cannot be obtained from the history and of course it is possible to have strongly positive skin tests to grass pollen without suffering from allergic disease at all. Neither allergy skin testing nor radioallergosorbent testing (RAST) nor measurement of total IgE is of any additional value in the diagnosis of seasonal allergic rhinitis and X-rays of the sinuses are not warranted. Investigations are needed, however, if the history is not consistent with seasonal episodes of running and itching of the eyes, nasal irritation, rhinorrhoea and nasal blockage. Persistent unilateral nasal obstruction warrants careful rhinoscopy to exclude the rare nasal tumours, and symptoms extending beyond the spring, summer and autumn do require further investigation to elicit important allergic causes such as household pets, the house dust mite and occupational factors for which useful avoidance therapy can be advocated.

TREATMENT

Decongestants

Inhalation of extracts of essential oils has been fashionable for the treatment of nasal congestion since Victorian times. Even today many people rely on lozenges and inhalations containing menthol, camphor and eucalyptus. Interestingly, although there is no evidence to show that these substances have any action on nasal blood vessels and therefore blockage, recent studies have shown that they have a definite central action increasing the sensation of nasal airflow. Vasoconstrictors are used by millions of hay fever sufferers worldwide and indeed their use is rooted in antiquity. Ephedrine is the active constituent of Ma Huang, a Chinese herbal medicine which has been used for more than 5000 years, and is still used today. All commercially available nasal vasoconstrictors possess adrenergic properties to a greater or lesser extent and cause contraction of the smooth muscle of the venous erectile tissue, thereby increasing nasal patency. Classical studies in the 1960s on the rabbit nasal mucosa showed that the effectiveness of such sympathomimetics varied in terms of time to onset, duration of

Table 1: Nasal decongestants

	Vaso-constrictor activity	Duration of action	Rapidity of action	Lack of reactive hyperaemia and tachyphylaxis
Noradrenaline	+	+	+ +	+
Adrenaline	+ +	+	+ + +	+
Xylometazoline	+ +	+ + +	+	+ + +
Oxymetazoline	+ +	+ + +	+	+ + +
Naphazoline	+ + +	+ +	+ +	+ +

action, vasoconstrictor activity, tachyphylaxis and the likelihood of subsequent reactive hyperaemia or rebound congestion. It can be seen from Table 1 why preparations containing xylometazoline (e.g. Otrivine) or naphazoline (e.g. Antistin-privine) are so popular since they are potent, long lasting and remain effective after prolonged use with low risk of rebound congestion, at least in the short term (up to two to four weeks treatment). Rhinitis medicamentosa may occur after excessive and prolonged use of decongestants and it is thought to be due to tissue hypoxaemia from reduced mucosal blood flow. Rhinitis medicamentosa does not occur when these compounds are administered orally, though this route of administration is associated with several disturbing unwanted effects including restlessness, nausea, vomiting, insomnia, headache, tachycardia, dysrhythmias, hypertension and angina, and is contraindicated in patients with cardiovascular disease, thyrotoxicosis and those taking monoamine oxidase inhibitors. Clinical trials have confirmed the efficacy of these compounds in topical or oral form irrespective of the cause of nasal blockage.

Nasal obstruction can also be influenced beneficially by exercise, nebulised saline and wetting agents such as propylene and polyethylene glycol. An alternative way of influencing nasal decongestion in allergic rhinitis is to antagonise the effect of mast cell-derived mediators and for this reason many nasal decongestants are combined with antihistamines as in Actifed tablets.

Antihistamines

It is over 50 years since the first antihistamine, phenbenzamine, was used successfully in humans. Since that time a plethora of drugs with anti H $_1$ activity have been introduced into clinical practice e.g.

Table 2: Antihistamines

	Duration of action	Specificity for H_1 receptors	Effect on cognitive function	Anti-inflammatory effects
Triprolidine ⎫	a few	+	+	NK
Terfenadine ⎭	hours	+ +	–	NK
Loratadine ⎫	up to	+ +	–	+
Azatadine ⎭	9 hours	+ +	–	NK
Cetirizine ⎫		+ +	–	(+)
Hydroxyzine ⎬	20-25	+	+	NK
Chlorpheniramine ⎭	hours	+	+ +	NK
Astemizole	19 days	+ +	–	NK

chlorpheniramine, triprolidine, promethazine and cycloheptadine (Table 2). Whilst all exhibit competitive H_1 receptor antagonism their potency in this respect is often weak, necessitating the use of large doses therapeutically. This would not in itself be a disadvantage were it not for the additional activities of many of these compounds leading to undesirable anticholinergic and sedative effects. This situation was transformed by the introduction of two new H_1 antagonists terfenadine and astemizole which had no detectable sedative or anticholinergic activity.

Another highly selective H_1 antagonist, cetirizine, has been extensively studied in the last two years. Its effectiveness in the management of both seasonal and perennial rhinitis has been proved in double blind placebo controlled studies. It is rapidly active (within 40 minutes) and its duration of effects is sufficiently long to allow once daily administration. Like astemizole and terfenadine, cetirizine has little effect on cognitive function. It may have additional antiinflammatory activity, particularly against eosinophils and neutrophils.

There is some evidence that a combination of H_1 and H_2 receptor antagonists is more effective in reducing histamine induced nasal congestion than either an H_1 or H_2 antagonist alone. At present however, there is no evidence to recommend this combination in clinical practice.

Anti-allergic preparations

Sodium cromoglycate (SCG) introduced in 1965 has no direct antihistaminic or smooth muscle relaxing properties. Despite intensive study its mode of action remains controversial though traditionally it is considered to act by "stabilising" mast cells. If this were indeed to be its mode of action this drug should be particularly useful for the treatment of allergic rhinitis. Its clinical efficacy in pollen induced rhinitis has been demonstrated in a large scale multicentre investigation in three American cities with comparable pollen seasons. This double blind study showed that a 4% aqueous solution of SCG effectively reduced sneezing, rhinorrhoea and perceived nasal congestion. Eye irritation was also reduced. Although better than placebo, administration of SCG only reduces overall symptom scores by between 30 and 50% and, like antihistamines, is more effective in relieving sneezing and rhinorrhoea than nasal obstruction. A recent double blind double dummy comparative study of twice daily terfenadine 60mg and sodium cromoglycate 4% solution sprayed into each nostril four times daily indicated that both drugs effectively relieved nasal symptoms other than congestion to a similar extent. Administration of SCG is without unwanted effects but patient compliance is limited by its short acting effect necessitating frequent topical administration up to six times daily.

Recently a drug with similar properties to SCG, nedocromil sodium, has been studied in allergic respiratory disease. Initial studies showed that this compound had a significantly greater effect than SCG in inhibiting IgE-mediated histamine release from mast cells recovered by broncho-alveolar lavage from the lungs of macaque monkeys. These histamine containing cells are thought to have characteristics similar to the "mucosal type" mast cells found in the nasal mucous membrane of man. This suggests that nedocromil should be more effective than SCG in the management of allergic rhinitis. Indeed it has been shown that nedocromil significantly inhibits not only sneezing and rhinorrhoea but also nasal obstruction following allergen provocation in man. Studies to date on the efficacy of this compound in seasonal allergic rhinitis are encouraging.

Anticholinergic preparations

Theoretically atropine ought to exhibit considerable benefit in the control of watery rhinorrhoea and viral induced rhinitis. However there are no placebo controlled trials which have proved its efficacy. Since atropine is readily absorbed there is a risk of systemic side effects. Ipratropium bromide, however, is only poorly absorbed from mucous membranes, and has been found to be of considerable value in the management of reversible airflow limitation occurring in the bronchi. High doses, up to 400µg four times a day, applied topically to the nasal mucosa have been shown to reduce rhinorrhoea but not sneezing or nasal blockage. Patients whose predominant symptom is that of profuse nasal discharge may well benefit from the use of this compound.

Corticosteroids

The widespread use of corticosteroid aerosols in the treatment of rhinitis began in the early 1970s with the introduction of beclomethasone dipropionate (BDP) which has a high local anti-inflammatory activity but substantial first pass metabolism in the liver greatly reducing its inhibitory effect on the hypothalamic pituitary axis (HPA).

Three synthetic corticosteroids are in common use for the topical treatment of rhinitis. Flunisolide is as potent but budesonide twice as potent as BDP in tests of antiinflammatory activity, an effect mirrored in clinical studies. Topical corticosteroids have been shown to be more efficacious than SCG in the control of nasal symptoms including obstruction in several double blind trials. In a double blind, double dummy comparative study of 61 adults with grass pollen induced rhinitis, twice daily treatment with budesonide (400µg) was superior to dexchlorpheniramine sustained release tablets (6mg b.d.) in relieving nasal obstruction, though the drugs were equally effective in controlling symptoms of sneeze and nasal discharge. However, the antihistamine tablets were more beneficial in the treatment of allergic conjunctivitis though they did cause drowsiness. The patients favoured the topical corticosteroids.

The introduction of the new non-sedative antihistamines has redressed the balance between treatment with antihistamines and topical corticosteroids in the management of rhinitis. In a general practice double blind, double dummy trial of astemizole 10mg o.m. and BDP 200µg b.d. over the hay fever season in Glasgow, no differences were detected between the two treatments in relation to the control of nasal symptoms.

Depot injections of the microcrystalline ester methyl-prednisolone-acetate (DepoMedrone®), equivalent to 100 mg of prednisolone, are widely used for the control of hay fever. Such injections probably suppress adrenal function for up to three weeks and in a few cases cause atrophy at the site of injection. They are however effective, particularly in the control of nasal obstruction. Although there are no controlled studies of tablets of prednisolone (5mg daily) in the management of seasonal or perennial rhinitis, many clinicians are favourably impressed by their beneficial effects. Although corticosteroids are effective in the control of allergic rhinitis their exact mode of action remains to be established. Several clinical studies have demonstrated that treatment of rhinitic patients with flunisolide (200µg daily dose) or budesonide (100 or 400µg daily dose) for one week or with BDP (400µg daily) for two weeks significantly reduces the immediate nasal response to allergen. Corticosteroids have not generally been shown to be effective in preventing the release of inflammatory mediators from mast cells although one study has demonstrated the ability of dexamethasone to inhibit the release of B-hexosaminidase, LTC_4 and LTB_4 from mouse bone marrow-derived mast cells. Treatment with topical corticosteroids such as BDP has, however, been shown to prevent the seasonal increase in the numbers of mast cells present in the nasal mucosa of rhinitic patients.

Treatment of rhinitic patients with flunisolide and BDP has also been shown, in some studies, to inhibit the late response to allergen. Corticosteroids have also been shown to reduce the sensitivity of irritant receptors and the secretory response to methacholine; actions which generally reduce the responsiveness of the nose in allergic rhinitis.

Drugs are now available which can control the symptoms of seasonal rhinitis in almost all patients. Unfortunately the majority of hay fever sufferers do not start their treatment until symptoms are well established. On theoretical grounds it is best to begin treatment before pollen is present in the atmosphere so preventing the development of inflammation in the nasal mucous membrane and probable "priming". In addition aerosol treatment can hardly be expected to be effective if airflow into the nostrils is negligible due to mucosal swelling. Under these circumstances vasoconstrictor nasal drops containing α-adrenoceptor agonists must be used to establish airflow prior to use of corticosteroid aerosols. It is vital that such drops are properly administered in the head down and forward position which has been shown to give optimal results.

BIBLIOGRAPHY

Angaard A, Malm L. Orally adminstered decongestant drugs in disorders of the upper respiratory passages. A survey of clinical results. *Clin Otolaryngol* 1984; **9**: 43–9.

Berman B, Buchman E, Dockhorn R, Leese P, Mansmann H, Middleton E. Cetirizine (C) therapy of perennial allergic rhinitis (PAR). *J Allergy Clin Immunol* 1988; **88**: 177.

Connell JT, Linzmayer I. Studies of rebound phenomena and oxymetazoline. *J Allergy Clin Immunol* 1988; **81**: 179.

Corrado OJ, Gomez E, Baldwin DL, Clague JE, Davies RJ. The effect of nedocromil sodium on nasal provocation with allergen. *J Allergy Clin Immunol* 1987; **80**: 218–22.

Davies RR, Smith LP. Weather and the grass pollen content of the air. *Clin Allergy* 1973; **3**: 95–108.

Emanuel MB. Hay fever, a post industrial revolution epidemic: a history of its growth during the 19th Century. *Clin Allergy* 1988; **18**: 295–304.

Fleming DM, Crombie DL. Prevalence of asthma and hay fever in England and Wales. *Br Med J* 1987; **294**: 279–83.

Gomez E, Corrado OJ, Baldwin DL, Swanston AR, Davies RJ. Direct in-vivo evidence for mast cell degranulation during allergen induced reaction in man. *J Allergy Clin Immunol* 1986; **78**: 637–45.

Handelman NI, Friday GA. Schwartz HJ, *et al.* Cromolyn sodium nasal solution in the prophylactic treatment of pollen-induced seasonal allergic rhinitis. *J Allergy Clin Immunol* 1977; **59**: 237– 42.

Howarth PH, Holgate ST. Comparative trial of two non-sedative H_1 antihistamines, terfenadine and astemizole for hay fever. *Thorax* 1984; **39**: 668–72.

Kershaw CR. Passive smoking, potential atopy and asthma in the first five years. *J Roy Soc Med* 1987; **80**: 683–8.

Kirkegaard J, Mygind N, Molgard F, *et al.* Ordinary and high-dose ipratropium in perennial non-allergic rhinitis. *J Allergy Clin Immunol* 1987; **79**: 585–90.

Naclerio RM, Meier HL, Kagey-Sobotka A, *et al.* Mediator release after nasal airway challenge with allergen. *Am Rev Resp Dis* 1983; **128**: 597–602.

Pipkorn U, Karlsson G, Enerback L. The cellular response of the human allergic mucosa to natural allergen exposure. *J Allergy Clin Immunol* 1988; **81**: 172.

Siegel SC, Katz R, Rachelefsky GS, *et al.* Multicentre study of beclomethasone dipropionate nasal aerosol in adults with seasonal allergic rhinitis. *J Allergy Clin Immunol* 1982; **69**: 345–53.

Viegas M, Gomez E, Brooks J, Davies RJ. The effect of the pollen season on nasal mast cell numbers. *Br Med J* 1987; **294**: 414.

Wood SF. Oral antihistamine or nasal steroid in hay fever: a double-blind double-dummy comparative study of once daily oral astemizole vs. twice daily nasal beclomethasone dipropionate. *Clin Allergy* 1986; **16**: 195–201.

Chapter 8

PERENNIAL RHINITIS

W. Franklin

Inflammation of the nasal mucosa occurs chronically or recurrently in a vast number of patients. It is estimated that allergic rhinitis affects about 10% of the population, thus making it the most common of the allergic diseases. In addition, many patients suffer similar symptoms without any evidence of allergy. These can be classified as having non-allergic or vasomotor rhinitis. In many patients with chronic rhinitis the diagnosis is missed and the problem is erroneously ascribed to infection. The diagnosis of sinusitis is made by the physician, or called "sinus" or "sinus trouble" by the patient. Sometimes symptoms are ascribed to recurrent "colds". Chronic nasal obstruction can also be attributed to anatomical abnormalities such as a deviated septum, when it may in fact be due to diffuse swelling of the mucous membranes.

This chapter emphasizes the clinical management of rhinitis and its aim is to be useful to the primary care physician. Allergic inflammation is discussed in more detail in Chapter 3. Diagnostic and therapeutic measures that are usually carried out by a specialist are discussed, chiefly to define their place in management. The reader who is interested in further detail is referred to excellent general texts on allergy [1, 2, 3], and to recent articles on the subject [4, 5].

Many classifications of rhinitis have been proposed. In Table 1 is a suggested classification. We prefer the term non-allergic rhinitis to vasomotor rhinitis because factors other than vasodilatation may be responsible for the oedema and inflammation. Because conjunctivitis is often present as well, many prefer the term rhinoconjunctivitis. It is more likely that conjunctivitis will be present when there is an allergic factor than when there is not. Conjunctivitis can exist, however, with the presence of nasal symptoms.

Non-allergic rhinitis is sometimes subdivided on the basis of the presence or absence of an eosinophilic exudate. The former has been labelled the NARES syndrome [6, 7].

Most patients do not fit neatly into one category or the other and have a combination of non-allergic rhinitis, which is the nasal analogue of intrinsic asthma, and allergic rhinitis, the nasal analogue of extrinsic asthma. The total number of patients with allergic rhinitis, non-allergic rhinitis, and those with symptoms that are not recognised as due to chronic rhinitis is huge, probably nearing forty million patients or 20% of the population of the United States [8]. There is no reason to believe that United States' experience differs from that of Europe or other industrialised nations.

The cause of non-allergic rhinitis is not known. Allergic rhinitis can be caused by seasonal allergens such as pollens and sometimes moulds. When symptoms are primarily seasonal, the term seasonal allergic rhinitis is often used. When substances such as dust, mites, feathers and animal danders cause perennial symptoms, the term perennial allergic rhinitis is used. However, most patients are allergic to both seasonal and perennial allergens and have perennial symptoms with or without seasonal exacerbations. A succession of seasonal allergens may mask any seasonality. Seasonal allergens and the aerobiology of such allergens are considered in the previous chapter.

SYMPTOMS

Nasal blockage, sneezing and nasal discharge are the major symptoms and can be continuous or intermittent. Sneezing is sometimes paroxysmal. Symptoms can be present separately or together. Often blockage and discharge alternate. Itching of the eyes, nose and palate are sometimes the chief complaint. Tearing, reddening of the conjunctivae and swelling of the eyelids can be prominent.

Table 1: Classification of rhinitis

	Based on presence of allergic factors	Other names
I.	Allergic rhinitis	Hay fever
		Seasonal rhinitis
		Perennial rhinitis
II.	Non-allergic rhinitis	Vasomotor rhinitis
	a. Eosinophilia	NARES
	b. Non-eosinophilic	
III.	Mixed rhinitis	

Headaches can occur even when there is only involvement of the nasal mucosa and no evidence of sinusitis. Pain is referred to the forehead; lateral to the nose; around the eyes; over the cheeks and sometimes the temple and vertical regions of the skull. Suppression of nasal inflammation by antihistaminics and topical steroids can relieve the headache. Because headache may be present without nasal blockage, discharge or sneezing, the role of rhinitis in causing the headache may not be recognized.

Decrease or loss of taste and smell are common. Careful questioning usually shows that it is smell rather than taste that is deficient. This is probably due to failure of odour-producing substances to reach the olfactory receptors because of oedema of the mucosa or polyps. Loss of smell often persists even after polypectomy.

Postnasal drip is a common symptom which is difficult to define and is often present without any physical evidence. Loss of hearing and earaches may be present due to eustachian tube dysfunction, which causes retraction and immobilisation of the ear drums.

Symptoms may be provoked by nonspecific factors such as strong odours, smoke, or changes in temperature or humidity. When allergic factors are present, exposure to allergens may be associated with a prompt flare-up of symptoms, but often the relationship is delayed and not perceived.

Many patients become dependent on the use of nasal vasoconstrictor drops or sprays and then develop what is known as rhinitis medicamentosa. Nasal congestion is a common occurrence during pregnancy and may occur in patients who otherwise are well.

Women with chronic rhinitis may worsen during pregnancy and improve after delivery. Asthma is present in about 50% of patients who have rhinitis, but in patients whose chief problem is asthma an even higher percentage have an associated rhinitis. The life pattern of the two syndromes in patients who ultimately suffer from both is also variable. Asthma in childhood often precedes rhinitis whereas in adults the reverse sequence is common.

PHYSICAL FINDINGS

Physical abnormalities are not the major feature of the disease. Symptoms usually outweigh the physical findings. Classically there is a pale, boggy, bluish nasal mucous membrane. Sometimes the pallor and swelling are striking but often deviation from average colour is minimal and in some cases the mucosa may even be redder than average. Nasal polyps are often present but may be obscured by a diffusely swollen mucosa. There is often reddening of the conjunctivae and swelling of the eyelids. So-called "allergic shiners" may be present. These are caused by trauma to small blood vessels in the eyelids. In extreme cases there may be oedema of the bulbar conjunctivae.

In many instances the patients will rub their noses in the typical "allergic salute" and repeated rubbing may cause a horizontal crease known as the "allergic crease".

PATHOGENESIS

Allergic inflammation has been discussed in Chapter 3. The nose acts as a filter which is especially effective with large particles such as pollen grains. This may account for the fact that pollen is a much more important cause of rhinitis than asthma. Small particles such as dust and dander may also be partially removed in the nose but a larger fraction escapes filtration in the nose and reaches the bronchial tree. The allergens in pollen are proteins on the outer surface, and play a role in the recognition of the appropriate pollen grain by the pistil on the female flower. These proteins are relatively soluble, penetrate the nasal mucosa and are capable of stimulating specific IgE production. They also react with mast cells bearing specific IgE to these same allergens. Degranulation of the mast cell occurs when two specific IgE molecules are joined by allergen. The granules contain chemical mediators which take part in allergic inflammation. Some of these mediators cause an immediate response and others cause reactions that are not manifest for four to 24 hours.

DIAGNOSIS

Unlike asthma, where in most cases, a tracing of forced expiration reflects the inflammatory changes, there is no simple readily reproducable test as useful in rhinitis. Rhinomanometry discussed in Chapter 4 and nasal peak flow rates [9] are not widely used for the diagnosis of nasal obstruction. Diagnosis depends on typical or at least consistent symptoms which are aggravated by factors which provoke or increase inflammation and which are relieved by

Table 2: Diagnosis of rhinitis

1. Consistent symptoms
   Nasal blockage
   Nasal discharge
   Sneezing
   Postnasal discharge
   Headache
   Loss of taste or smell
   Postnasal discharge
   Ear blockage
2. Physical findings
   Swelling of mucosa and turbinates
   Pallor of mucosa and turbinates
   Polyps
   Mucoid exudate
3. Response to therapy with one or more of the following:
   Antihistaminics
   Adrenergic agents
   Topical steroids
   Systemic steroids

measures which decrease inflammation (Table 2). The history alone may be sufficient. Typical symptoms such as sneezing and discharge of blockage which wax and wane in relation to season, place, or clear-cut exposure not only confirm the diagnosis of rhinitis but also suggest an allergic cause. When symptoms are constant or exacerbate for no apparent reason, the response to treatment with antihistaminics, decongestants or topical steroids separately or in combination confirms the diagnosis. A therapeutic test is essential when symptoms are atypical. Headache may be the only complaint, but a clear cut therapeutic response suggests that the headache is in fact a referred sensation from an inflamed nasal mucosa. Worsening and improvement as medication is withdrawn and reinstituted confirms the diagnosis. Sometimes topical steroids are ineffective because they do not reach the site of inflammation. This is particularly true when the chief complaint is earache or loss of smell. These symptoms arise because of swelling outside of the airstream. Deposition of topical steroids is then inadequate. Although the continued use of systemic steroids is rarely justified in rhinitis, a therapeutic test of several days to a few weeks may define the problem.

Blood eosinophilia is often present in rhinitis but is not as striking as in asthma. A normal eosinophil count does not rule out the diagnosis of rhinitis. An elevated eosinophil count may occur both in the presence or absence of specific allergic factors and suggests that steroids will be effective.

Examination of nasal or conjunctival smears present the same problem of defining the sample as does examination of the sputum, but sometimes such studies are helpful in recognising an eosinophilic inflammatory process.

X-ray examination of the nasal sinuses is chiefly of value in detecting associated sinus disease. However, it is often difficult to be certain on the basis of X-ray changes alone that sinus infection is present. Thickening of the basement membrane can occur without infection. Clouding of the sinuses may be due to polypoid changes. Presence of a fluid level, however, strongly suggests infection. Even when sinusitis is present, it does not mean that diffuse rhinitis is not the cause of much of the patient's complaint. Other anatomical changes such as a deviated septum may also not account for the patient's complaint, and the contribution of infection or diffuse rhinitis to airway obstruction may only be apparent after each process is treated.

Differential diagnosis

The chief problem is to decide when infection rather than non-infectious nasal inflammation is the cause of symptoms. Patients and their doctors often attribute symptoms to upper respiratory infections or ''colds''. It is sometimes impossible to decide whether an upper respiratory infection is present in someone who has recurrent nasal discharge, blockage and sneezing. It is not likely, however, that patients who are otherwise well would suffer more than three or four ''colds'' per year or that they would have colds lasting more than a week or two at a time. Both frequency and duration of symptoms become major differentiating points. Frequent or prolonged episodes should lead to a consideration of allergic factors, tests for eosinophilia, and most importantly, a therapeutic test with antihistaminics, alpha adrenergic agents and steroids rather than the recurrent use of antibiotics. To be sure, these agents may also have some effect on viral upper respiratory infections but do not alter the course of the illness as dramatically as in chronic rhinitis. The criteria for making a presumptive diagnosis of chronic rhinitis are given in Table 2 and the chief differential diagnoses to be considered are listed in Table 3.

A question commonly asked by ENT specialists and primary care

Table 3: Differential diagnosis of chronic rhinitis

1.	Upper respiratory infection—"colds"
2.	Sinusitis
3.	Deviated septum
4.	Other causes of headache
5.	Rhinitis of pregnancy
6.	Antihypertensive drugs
7.	Immunodeficiency
8.	Myxoedema
9.	Nasal vasoconstrictor abuse

Table 4: Rhinitis: complications and associated conditions

1.	Otitis media
2.	Sinusitis
3.	Nasal polyps
4.	Asthma

physicians is "Does allergy play a role in causing recurrent otitis or sinusitis?" A more appropriate question is "Does the patient have chronic rhinitis as a contributory cause of these problems" and if the answer is positive, "Does allergy play a role in causing the rhinitis?"

COMPLICATIONS AND ASSOCIATED CONDITIONS

Complications are listed in Table 4. There is no question that recurrent sinusitis and recurrent otitis are common with people who have chronic rhinitis. Almost all patients who have polyps also have chronic diffuse inflammation of the nasal mucous membrane. Asthma is commonly associated with rhinitis and probably represents inflammation of the lower airway caused by the same factors that are producing inflammation in the nose. Cough is a common symptom in rhinitis. It has been attributed to a reflex mechanism stimulated by nasal and sinus inflammation and postnasal drip but may in fact represent an extension of the inflammatory process down to the trachea and larger bronchi, where the cough receptors are most numerous.

Nasal polyps are discussed in the next chapter. Nasal polyps are often associated with asthma and aspirin sensitivity in the so-called "classic triad". However aspirin sensitivity can be present without either polyps or asthma. Patients often have long standing rhinitis before aspirin sensitivity becomes apparent. The mechanism of the adverse reaction to aspirin is poorly understood, but probably involves an abnormality in the metabolism of arachidonic acid. Patients often suffer flare ups of rhinitis or asthma with other non-steroidal antiinflammatory drugs, but can tolerate acetaminophen and sodium salicylate [10].

DIAGNOSIS OF ALLERGIC FACTORS

Allergic factors are probably present in more than half of the patients who present with the symptoms of rhinitis. The main means of detecting these factors are summarised in Table 5.

Table 5: Diagnosis of allergic factors

1. History
2. Skin tests—RAST
3. Total IgE
4. Elimination

History

The history is the major diagnostic tool in recognising allergy as a cause of rhinitis. A high degree of seasonality suggests the role of pollens, or even in some cases seasonal exposure to moulds or mites. The role of substances that are not constantly present in the environment may be recognised by the patient. Sometimes symptoms are worse in a particular place or improve when the patient leaves his or her usual environment such as the home or workplace. Such relationships may direct attention to household pets, carpets, occupational allergens, or mouldy ventilation systems. On the other hand, substances constantly in the environment may go unrecognised. One may be forced to make a presumptive diagnosis of the role of such substances based on a consistent history and a positive skin reaction. This is often true of the major cause of perennial rhinitis, the house dust mite, and is also true of moulds. Most patients with allergic rhinitis have multiple sensitivities. Even though they may be allergic to seasonal substances such as pollens, non-seasonal or perennial symptoms may result from a succession of pollen seasons, or a combination of mite and pollen sensitivity. The causative role of any one substance may not be definable by the history.

Skin tests

The only recognised mechanism by which environmental allergens cause rhinitis and asthma involves IgE specific for the allergen. Therefore, a demonstration of specific IgE is needed for a diagnosis of allergic rhinitis. Although such a demonstration is necessary, it is not sufficient because many patients have specific IgE to substances that clearly do not cause symptoms under the usual conditions of exposure. On the other hand, failure to demonstrate specific IgE to a substance probably means that it does not play a role in causing symptoms.

The best way of demonstrating specific IgE is the skin test (see Chapter 3). It must be emphasised that skin tests must not be done when skin reactivity is being suppressed by antihistaminic drugs which are usually the mainstay of symptomatic treatment in rhinitis. It is necessary to maintain potent extracts. Standardisation is a problem because allergens deteriorate rapidly in solution and therefore it is difficult for physicians who do not do many skin tests to maintain potent testing materials. Prick tests are easier and safer to perform than intracutaneous tests. Many allergists believe that prick tests are adequate for the diagnosis of clinical allergy. This may be true for highly potent allergens such as pollens, but is clearly not true of many patients who are allergic to mites, feathers, and animal danders.

Unless positive reactions to a perennial allergen can be demonstrated, it is difficult to ascribe perennial symptoms to allergic mechanisms alone. If the patient has skin reactivity only to seasonal pollens but has perennial symptoms, one may have to conclude that the patient is suffering from a combination of allergic and non-allergic rhinitis. It is also possible that the patient has only non-allergic rhinitis and that the skin reactions are irrelevant. It is often difficult to resolve this issue.

The radioallergosorbent test, or RAST, is widely used as a means of detecting specific IgE. This has been discussed in Chapter 3. Since it is less sensitive and more expensive than the skin test, the indications for using it are few. Generalized rash is not common in patients whose chief problem is rhinitis and most patients with rhinitis can forego antihistaminics long enough to permit adequate skin testing.

Not every patient who has the symptoms of rhinitis needs to be tested, but if symptoms are not trivial or require the continued use of medication, an attempt should be made to define and deal with

Table 6: Extracts for testing

Mites
Dust
Cat dander
Dog dander
Feathers
Major pollens:
Grass—Timothy, others
Trees—Birch, oak
Weeds—Ragweed, sage
Moulds:
Alternaria, Hormodendron, Penicillium, Aspergillus

allergic causes. Negative skin tests mean that the patient does not have a significant amount of specific IgE for the allergens tested and usually means that one is dealing with non-allergic rhinitis. Such a conclusion is warranted, however, only if a battery of skin tests is done which includes all of the major inhalant allergens. It is probably not necessary to do more than two or three dozen tests in evaluating perennial rhinitis and one could probably recognize allergic factors adequately if one tested with the extracts listed in Table 6. Foods are almost never the cause of rhinitis.

Total IgE

Tests of total serum IgE are performed by laboratories that serve most physicians' offices. Although it would seem logical to use such a test as an index of the presence of specific IgE, it is usually not clinically useful. Many patients who give a history of clear cut clinical sensitivity and who have striking skin reactions to one or more relevant allergens have total IgE levels which are well within the normal range. Thus doing a total IgE does not help one to decide whether or not to proceed with skin tests. Furthermore, when skin tests are negative, one rarely finds an elevated level of IgE that would suggest tests other than those included in the standard battery should be carried out.

Eosinophilia

Eosinophilia in the blood and in the nasal smear have been discussed already in this chapter. Contrary to common belief, eosinophilia does help distinguish between allergic and non-allergic rhinitis [7].

Elimination

When the history does not help one decide whether a substance that produces a positive skin reaction is clinically relevant, one can sometimes make the decision by eliminating the substance from the environment. Feather pillows, reservoirs of mites such as bedroom rugs or animals can be temporarily removed. Sometimes it is easier to remove the patient from the environment. A fully carpeted home or one with several animals may be better evaluated in this manner. Often, however, exposure to dust, mites, and danders cannot be sufficiently lessened to enable one to observe a significant reduction in symptoms.

Challenge

Instillation of allergenic extracts into the eye or into the nasal passages can produce symptoms or observable changes in the nasal mucosa such as swelling, erythema, or pallor. There can also be a change in nasal airway resistance which can be measured by rhinomanometry. Chemical inhibitors of allergic inflammations are released into the nasal secretions [11]. Such challenges have often been used as a research tool to study allergic reactions and to demonstrate the effect of treatment with drugs or immunotherapy. This approach is time consuming and not cost effective in clinical management. Furthermore, exposure differs significantly from that which occurs naturally and tests may be difficult to perform in patients with ongoing symptoms. Most importantly, even though a patient may develop symptoms on challenge, it does not prove that the substance in question is the major cause of the symptoms which brought the patient to the physician. The patient's symptoms may be primarily due to some other allergen or even due primarily to nonallergic rhinitis. Therefore challenges are rarely carried out in the clinical evaluation of patients.

ENVIRONMENTAL CONTROLS

When evidence suggests that allergens cause symptoms, the first approach should be to reduce exposure.

Even when specific allergens cannot be incriminated in the common allergic syndromes, environmental factors may play a role.

Irritating dust, fumes, smoke and gases, humidity, cold air, and strong odours may provoke symptoms. Certain measures which are of great importance are often neglected in the management of patients. On the other hand, burdening the patient with a long litany of recommendations may lead to failure to carry out the few changes that are indeed important.

Non specific factors

Humidity There is a controversy regarding the role of humidity in aggravating the symptoms of rhinitis and asthma. Many claim that humidifiers benefit symptoms such as cough, postnasal drip, and dryness of the nasal membranes. On the other hand, patients often do well in a dry climate, perhaps because exposure to mites and mould is reduced. Furthermore, humidifiers themselves can be the source of important allergens such as moulds and can promote the growth of mites. In cold climates during the winter it is almost impossible to increase the humidity of heated indoor air without causing outside walls and windows to be dripping wet. We therefore do not encourage the use of humidifiers unless the patient notes symptomatic improvement, and generally advise avoidance of humidifiers when patients are allergic to dust, mites or moulds.

Temperature Indoor temperatures are usually not extreme enough to warrant attention in most instances. On the other hand, certain occupations such as work in refrigerators or activities such as exercise in the cold air may be worth restricting. Cold air clearly provokes rhinorrhoea.

Irritants Ammonia, chlorine, soap powder, smoke from cigarettes and wood stoves can aggravate both asthma and rhinitis. Cigarette smoke is a particularly potent factor, but prohibition of smoking by both the patient and by other members of the household is a goal that is often difficult to achieve. The physician should unequivocally support efforts to rid the house and work environments of tobacco smoke. In recent years, the law in the United States has been helpful and smoking in offices, restaurants and other public areas is becoming more limited. The physician should be prepared to support the patient if a legal approach becomes necessary. Unfortunately less attention is given to smoking in Europe and Asia.

Small houses and mobile homes with formaldehyde insulation

may have a high enough formaldehyde concentration to be irritating. However, this is often blamed for symptoms when levels are not high, and when symptoms are not typical of any known syndrome. The odour of paint, especially oil-based, is a common aggravating factor. Patients may have to move out while their house is being painted. Insecticides, which are often cholinesterase inhibitors, may produce a variety of symptoms which may include systemic and gastrointestinal symptoms as well as respiratory symptoms.

Control of allergens

Avoidance of allergens is often possible but sometimes requires an unacceptable change in lifestyle. The efficacy of measures short of total removal of a source of allergen such as a dog, cat, or feather pillow has been based on the assumption that some of the measures make sense. Immunochemical techniques for determining the amount of allergen in air samples taken from the patient's environment are being developed. It will soon be possible to define the benefit to be derived from such manoeuvres as getting rid of a carpet, encasing a mattress, or restricting an animal.

Since most allergens are particulate, they can be removed from the air by settling or by air cleaners. Settling of particles is especially important for particles as large as whole pollen grains or mould spores. Particles settle according to Stoke's Law:

$$V_t = \frac{density \times g \times diameter^2}{18 \times air\ viscosity}$$

V_t is the terminal velocity. At ordinary temperatures and pressures $V_t = 2.9 \times 10^5 \times density \times diameter^2$ (cm/sec). Since most particles are of approximately unit density, Table 7 indicates the terminal velocity for various size particles of unit density and the time to clear an average 8 ft high room.

Thus most large particles, even particles down to the size that can be retained in the lung, are cleared by settling within a few hours if not repeatedly reintroduced into the environment. Air cleaners therefore may not be necessary if the source or reservoir of allergens is removed.

Air cleaners can remove air particles down to 0.3 μm or less in

Table 7: Settling of particles[a]

Diameter (μ)	V_t (cm/sec)	Time to clear 244 cm (8 ft)
40	4.8	51 sec
20	1.2	3 min 20 sec
10	0.29	7 min
6	0.11	37 min
4	0.05	1 hour 21 min
2	0.013	5.2 hours
1	0.0003	22.6 hours

[a] For spherical particles of unit density. V_t = terminal velocity.

diameter. Thus some viruses, fumes and smoke can be removed. Effective air cleaners are of two types: mechanical filters and electrostatic filters. Mechanical filters are easier to maintain because the filters can be changed. In order to be effective, however, pore size must be small and the resistance to air flow great. Such filters are called high efficiency particle arrester or HEPA. Air flow resistance limits the area of efficacy unless an inordinate amount of power is expended. While this approach seems rational there are few studies to show efficacy [12]. Furthermore, one would not expect a patient's total exposure for a ubiquitous substance such as dust to be substantially reduced unless the patient is breathing cleaned air most of the time. An air cleaner blowing air at the patient's pillow or at an office desk may have substantial impact. However, a highly efficient device at the opposite end of the room with a large rug in between *may* have little impact on the patient's exposure.

Recommendations for specific allergens

Pollens Pollens are the major cause of seasonal rhinitis but can aggravate perennial rhinitis. A major impact on pollen exposure can be made by staying indoors during the pollen season. A room air conditioner which recirculates air will soon permit the room to be pollen free if the windows are kept closed. A highly efficient filter is not needed. When the weather is cool merely keeping the windows shut will achieve the same result.

Driving a car with the windows closed will also reduce exposure. Long drives through the countryside during the pollen season should be avoided, as should outside activities such as picnics and golf. Seashore activity if the prevailing wind is off the sea may be substituted. Lawn mowing will produce heavy concentrations of pollen and mould. Exposure is not limited to grass pollen. Tree pollens descend on the grass and are disseminated when the lawn is mowed.

Sometimes local conditions are important. A large tree outside a patio may produce overwhelming concentrations of pollen. Fields of grass upwind from a home may have to be mowed before the grass pollinates.

Moulds Mould spores can be produced indoors as well as outdoors. Outdoor moulds can be excluded by keeping the windows closed. Indoor moulds may be a problem when there is excessive moisture. Damp basements, especially if there is a dirt floor, can produce large amounts of indoor mould. Such conditions may require major alteration in the house or a change of residence. Dehumidifiers may be helpful. Efficacy of antifungal agents is not clear. Although moulds grow in flower pots, there is little dissemination of spores from this source and therefore house plants do not have to be excluded from the house.

Animals Since the most common identifiable cause of asthma is animal dander every effort should be made to convince patients who react to animal dander to get rid of household pets. Many patients and their families, however, will not accept this recommendation, but will accept lesser measures. Patients often deny the role of a beloved pet because exposure may have preceded the illness, a common sequence of events, because sensitisation may require years of exposure. On the other hand, they sometimes argue the reverse because symptoms due initially to other allergens preceded getting the pet. They may fail to observe a relationship between exposure and symptoms unless exposure stops for weeks at a time. Animals should at least be excluded from the bedroom and other areas of the home where the patient spends a great deal of time, even when the patient is not at home. Carpets are reservoirs of dander as well as mites. Rooms that are carpeted retain dander for much longer periods than rooms with bare floors. It is difficult to stop children from petting and fondling animals so that getting rid of pets may be easier than constant nagging to reduce exposure.

If a hot air heating system is present, dander will be picked up from one area of the house where the pet is permitted and scattered throughout the rest of the house. Thus measures short of complete removal of pets often fail.

Dust and mites   The most important allergens in house dust are the mites *Dermatophygoides pteronyssinus* and *Dermatophygoides farinae*. Since dust and mites are ubiquitous and cannot be totally eliminated it may not be possible to define their role in causing symptoms. However, it is safer to presume that mites are clinically relevant in patients reacting by skin tests, and measures to reduce exposure should be carried out whether or not immunotherapy is also used [13]. Mites live in carpeting, bedding, mattresses and upholstered furniture and feed on human skin scales. Optimal conditions for growth are a temperature of about 70°F and 70% relative humidity. In the northern United States, interiors of houses are dry during the long heating season. This tends to kill mites but mite allergens may persist through the year even after the number of live mites decrease.

A major reservoir of dust, mites and dander is carpeting. Rooms that are carpeted have much more dust in the air than bare rooms because each time a rug is stepped on up comes an invisible cloud of dust which then takes minutes to hours to resettle. This does not happen if the floor has a hard surface such as wood or plastic. Vacuum cleaning and steam cleaning do not adequately reduce the burden of mites and other allergens. The best solution is to have a bare floor.

Mattresses should be covered with an impermeable encasing to seal in dust and mites. Surfaces can be sponged. All bedding outside of this cover should be washable and laundered in hot water (greater than 130°F) once a week. Prolonged drying (greater than four hours) at 140°F may be a substitute.

Feather filled pillows and comforters are not only bad for those allergic to feathers, but are potent sources of mites. Synthetic pillows should be used and washed frequently in hot water.

Upholstered furniture should be kept at a minimum and excluded from the bedroom.

Effective anti-mite agents (Acaricides) are not yet available and may not be practical because of the need for frequent use and potential toxicity. Some agents which may be of value are in the process of development.

Since most patients spend more time in their bedroom than in any other room of the house, particular attention should be paid to it. Furthermore, patients and families are more willing to remove a bedroom carpet than a living room carpet and to alter bedroom furnishings. If only one room is to be shielded from outside pollen by using a room air conditioner and keeping the window closed it should be the bedroom. In some instances, offices and studies should receive similar attention.

When there is a hot air heating system, dust, mites, dander and other allergens from other areas of the house can be introduced into the bedroom via the hot air ducts even though the bedroom itself has been dealt with meticulously. One can close off the hot air supply and heat the room with an electric heater. In some instances a study, a playroom or an office deserves as close attention as the bedroom.

Summary

A limited number of approaches to the environment are probably effective in reducing the symptoms of some of the common allergic syndromes. These are tabulated in Table 8. The importance of each measure depends on the patient's sensitivities and the patient's lifestyle. The more important changes should be stressed rather than burdening the patient with a long list of tasks that may have trivial impact. The most important of these are removal of pets, feathers and carpeting.

Table 8: Summary of environmental control

General measures	
1.	Humidity control—keep relative humidity at 50% or less
2.	Eliminate irritants, especially cigarette smoke, from home
Specific measures	
1.	Remove household pets
2.	Remove feathers—pillows, comforters, down jackets, birds
3.	Minimise carpeting—none in bedrooms
4.	Isolate patient's bedroom from hot air heating system
5.	Cover mattress with dust-tight encasing. Launder bedding and pillows in hot water regularly (every 1–4 weeks)
6.	Windows closed during pollen season
7.	Air condition bedroom and car

IMMUNOTHERAPY

Injections of grass pollen extract were first reported to be effective in hayfever over 75 years ago [14]. The premise that specific, but generally harmless, substances in the environment caused symptoms in susceptible individuals and that injections of extracts of these substances over a long period of time would alleviate

Table 9: Characteristics of a good controlled study of immunotherapy

1.	Selection of sensitive cases
2.	Random assignment
3.	Placebo control
4.	Blind evaluation
5.	Adequate dosage
6.	Sensitive index of response
7.	Adequate statistical analysis

symptoms became widely held before specific IgE and IgG were recognised as factors in the process. At first, this approach was called desensitisation, but when it became clear that skin reactivity was not depleted by the process, the term hyposensitisation was substituted. We now recognise the possible role of specific IgG blocking antibodies, and regulatory T cells, and the failure of clinical response to correlate well with any immunological parameter. The term immunotherapy does not commit itself to which immunological mechanism may be responsible for clinical response and is therefore more appropriate.

During the first half of this century no adequately controlled studies of this form of treatment were carried out. Based on uncontrolled observations of patients, however, using the patient's recollections of the past as a comparison, a consensus was formed which may be termed "standard immunotherapy." This may be briefly stated as follows: treatment to tolerance with extracts of pollens, dust and moulds over a period of months was effective in both allergic rhinitis and asthma.

Controlled studies of immunotherapy have been reviewed by the author [15]. A good controlled study should fulfill the criteria shown in Table 9.

Selection of sensitive cases is much easier in seasonal rhinitis than in perennial rhinitis, because the seasonality itself confirms the relevance of a seasonal allergen in patients selected on the basis of a positive skin reaction. At least 17 studies that fulfil the above criteria show clinical efficacy in rhinitis. Sixteen of these studies were done with seasonal allergens. In one study [15] showing efficacy with mite extract, patients were selected because they had asthma, a positive skin reaction to mite extract and a positive bronchial challenge with mite extract. Nevertheless 90% of these patients also had rhinitis which was improved by immunotherapy with mite extract.

The immunological changes that occur in the course of immunotherapy have been well reviewed [16]. These include development of specific IgG which may act as a blocking antibody. There is a long term decrease in the production of specific IgE, and changes in T lymphocytes responding to the allergen have been noted. Whether any or all of these changes are important to the clinical response is not clear.

There is no reason to believe that the clinical and immunological changes which have been observed in response to treatment with a single allergen would be different in patients who have perennial rhinitis and multiple sensitivities and are treated with several allergens. Clinical experience strongly favours such an approach.

The decision as to whether to initiate immunotherapy at all will depend on how hard it is to control the patient's symptoms with other measures. The nuisance and expense of rhinitis without immunotherapy must be balanced against the nuisance and expense of the immunotherapy. Further, in order for immunotherapy to be effective, a significant portion of the patient's symptoms must depend on allergic factors. This is often difficult to establish in perennial rhinitis. One may often settle for a presumptive diagnosis based on consistent symptoms and positive skin reactions. Once the decision is made to institute immunotherapy we believe that all major allergens to which the patient reacts by skin test and which are present in the patient's environment should be included in the treatment programme. This usually includes extracts of mites and dust, but may also include pollens and moulds. Treatment with animal dander extracts may also be indicated when exposure cannot be avoided. Even when the patient is willing to remove animals from his or her home, repeated exposure may be impossible to avoid without making the patient a social outcast.

Because of fatal reactions following injections of allergenic extracts, immunotherapy has been virtually discontinued in the UK. Such reactions are extremely rare and usually occur when this form of treatment is administered by non-specialists. The rest of the world continues to use this approach.

MEDICAL MANAGEMENT

Some of the agents used in the medical management of rhinitis are discussed in detail elsewhere and therefore in this chapter we will only summarise the place of medical management. Drug therapy is indicated whether rhinitis is allergic or non-allergic and whether symptoms are perennial or seasonal. Often a simple regimen is so

Table 10: Stepped care of rhinitis

Direct measures	
1.	Oral antihistaminics
2.	Oral adrenergic agents
3.	Topical antihistaminics and adrenergic agents to eye
4.	Topical nasal steroids
5.	Topical nasal cromolyn
6.	Topical cromolyn to eye
7.	Systemic steroids
Other measures	
1.	Antibiotics
2.	Saline irrigation

effective that further measures are unnecessary. This is especially true with seasonal rhinitis but even in perennial rhinitis many patients may elect to take medication most of the time rather than make major changes in their environment or undertake the burden of a prolonged programme of immunotherapy.

The stepped care of rhinitis is given in Table 10. Most physicians will start with antihistaminics with or without the addition of an adrenergic drug. Chlorpheniramine, brompheniramine, diphenhydramine, tripelennamine are all available over the counter in the United States, as are adrenergic agents such as phenylephrine and pseudoephedrine. The use of adrenergic agents topically can lead to rebound congestion, and the continued use leads to chronic inflammation known as rhinitis medicamentosa. Antihistaminics and adrenergic agents can be taken separately or in combination. Most patients will have tried these drugs before they come to a physician and are therefore seeking either more effective treatment or an antihistaminic that does not make them sleepy. When the latter is true, it is often possible to relieve their symptoms with terfenadine without making them drowsy. Many of the patients who come to a specialist, however, have already been given the measures described above and may even have been given topical steroids or cromolyn. Often the dose or technique of administration of these last two agents has been inadequate or the tempo of response has not been adequately explained and the patient gives up in the belief that such measures are ineffective. Retreatment with these agents using proper techniques often is effective.

The use of topical steroids over cromolyn is preferred because it is more effective in most patients, and works in a few days rather than weeks. By the time patients reach this point, they are most anxious for symptomatic relief. At a later date, after symptoms have been controlled, it may be possible to reduce the need for topical steroids, if one uses cromolyn topically. However, this is rarely effective enough to justify the nuisance.

In the United States metered dose inhalers of dexamethasone phosphate and beclomethasone dipropionate are available. Flunisolide in aqueous solution and beclomethasone dipropionate in a liquid suspension are also available in spray bottles. The adaptor currently available in the United States for beclomethasone dipropionate metered dose inhaler is too short and causes difficulties directing the aerosol [the manufacturer is understood to be modifying the adapter. Ed.]. Many find dexamethasone phosphate more effective and prefer to use it even though it is not inactivated after absorption and does cause some adrenal suppression. Flunisolide solution causes nasal stinging. This can be avoided by the use of beclomethasone dipropionate suspension (Beconase AQ or Vancenase AQ). This has become the best approach to the topical administration of steroids.

Although the continued use of systemic steroids in rhinitis is rarely justified, it is sometimes necessary to use systemic steroids initially because the nose is so swollen that topical steroids cannot effectively reach the nasal mucosa. When this is done, it is better to give steroids daily in divided doses rather than as a single AM dose or as a dose given on alternate days. The major place of systemic steroids in the management of rhinitis is for initial clearing of the nose so that topical measures can be effective, but occasionally systemic steroids are also given for diagnostic purposes. When symptoms are atypical and consist mainly of headache, ear blockage, loss of taste or smell or postnasal drip without concomitant discharge, sneezing, or nasal blockage, a therapeutic trial of systemic steroids may be effective and topical steroids alone may fail. Such an effect proves that the symptoms in question are based on a reversible inflammatory process. Treatment should not be continued any longer than is necessary to decide if the symptoms are reversible or not.

In the extremely rare instance where nasal blockage cannot be handled with topical steroids alone then an alternate day regimen of steroids may be justified.

Many patients may complain of dryness and crusting of the nasal mucosa either as part of the disease itself or as the result of treatment with antihistaminics or topical steroids. When this is the case physiological saline instilled into the nose can be helpful.

Infection is often difficult to recognise in the presence of a process that may be characterised by nasal discharge which is sometimes purulent in appearance because of the presence of eosinophils or other inflammatory cells. It may be necessary to give antibiotics. This often has to be done on an empirical basis because the organisms in the discharge may not reflect the true infecting agent.

Often mycoplasma rather than bacteria may be responsible for a flare-up. Erythromycin is a good drug to use in such situations but when bacterial infection is suspected, one of the penicillins may be the agent of choice. Sinus X-rays are sometimes helpful when making the decision as to whether a prolonged course of antibiotics should be given. An elevated total white blood count sometimes helps decide that this approach is correct, but often a decision is made on the basis of clinical response.

Perennial rhinitis is a chronic condition and the patient must be taught that some of the measures which are effective may have to be continued indefinitely. However, the need for medication waxes and wanes and one should always try to minimise the dose that will keep the patient comfortable without producing serious side effects. Most patients may initially require the standard dose of inhalations of a topical steroid and then can gradually reduce the dose to half that number of inhalations or less for long term maintenance.

SUMMARY

Nasal blockage, nasal discharge, sneezing, headache, earache and loss of taste and smell, symptoms responsible for many visits to primary care physicians, are commonly caused by chronic rhinitis, a non-infectious inflammation of the nasal mucosa. Inflammation can be caused by both allergic and non-allergic mechanisms. It is important to recognise the role of this kind of inflammation in causing symptoms, and not erroneously attribute symptoms to infection or anatomical abnormalities.

Diagnosis depends primarily on the response of the symptoms to treatment with antihistaminic drugs, adrenergic agents and corticosteroids. Although infection is not the prime cause of this syndrome, superimposed infections may require the use of antibiotics in addition to drugs which reduce swelling of the nasal mucosa.

Allergy plays a causative role in a large fraction of patients with rhinitis. The causative allergens are usually substances that are inhaled such as pollens, dust, mites, moulds and animal dander. Foods rarely cause rhinitis. The recognition of allergic causes depends on both the history and tests for specific IgE, the most sensitive of which is the skin test.

In perennial rhinitis as opposed to seasonal rhinitis, the history may fail to identify the causative role of substances constantly in the environment. Sometimes the suspect substance can be eliminated and the diagnosis confirmed. The effect of these substances can be reduced by changes in the environment and by immunotherapy with extracts of the causative allergens. Such measures, though often highly effective, are burdensome and expensive, and may not be necessary because medical management is usually safe and adequate to control symptoms.

REFERENCES

1. Patterson R, ed. *Allergic diseases: Diagnosis and management*, 3rd ed. Philadelphia: J. B. Lippincott, 1985.
2. Kaplan AP, ed. *Allergy*. New York: Churchill Livingstone, 1985.
3. Middleton E, Reed CE, Ellis EF, eds. *Allergy: Principles and practice*, 2nd ed. St Louis: CV Mosby, 1983.
4. Kaliner M, Eggleston PA, Matthews KP. Rhinitis and asthma. *JAMA* 1987; **258**: 2851–73.
5. Druce HM, Kaliner M. Allergic rhinitis. *JAMA* 1988; **259** : 260–3.
6. Jacobs RC, Freedman PM, Boswell RN. Nonallergic rhinitis with eosinophilia (NARES syndrome). *J Allergy Clin Immunol* 1981; **67**: 253.
7. Mullarkey MF, Hill J, Webb DR. Allergic and nonallergic rhinitis: their characteristics with attention to the meaning of nasal eosinophilia. *J Allergy Clin Immunol* 1980; **65**: 122.
8. National Institute of Allergy and Infectious Diseases Task Force Report. *NIAD: Asthma and other allergic diseases*. Bethesda: NIH publications 1979: 79–307.
9. Matthews KP. Allergic and nonallergic rhinitis, nasal polyposis and sinusitis immunology In: Kaplan AD, ed. *Allergy*. New York: Churchill Livingstone, 1985.
10. Stevenson DD. Adverse reactons to aspirin and nonsteroidal anti-inflammatory drugs; In: Reed CE, Bellanti J, Davies RJ, *et al*, eds. *Proceedings of the XII International Congress of Allergology and Clinical Immunology*. St Louis 1986: 79–83.
11. Naclerio RM, Proud D, Togias AG, *et al*. Inflammatory mediators in late antigen-induced rhinitis. *N Engl J Med* 1985; **313**: 65–70.
12. Nelson HS, Hirsch SR, Ohman JL, *et al*. Recommendations for the use of residential air-cleaning devices in the treatment of allergic respiratory disease. *J Allergy Clin Immunol* 1988; **82**: 661–9.
13. Platts-Mills TAE, Chapman MD. Dust mites: immunology, allergic disease and environmental control. *J Allergy Clin Immunol* 1987; **80**: 255–75.
14. Noon L. Prophylactic inoculation against hay fever. *Lancet* 1911; **i**: 1572.
15. Franklin W. Controlled studies of immunotherapy in allergic rhinitis: A critical

revies. In: Settipane GA, ed. *Rhinitis*. Providence, New England and Regional Allergy Proceedings 1984: 119–25.
16. Warner JO, Soothill JF, Price JF, Hay EN. Controlled trial of hyposensitizations to dermatophagoides pteronyssinus in children with asthma. *Lancet* 1978; **2**: 912.
17. Rocklin RE. Clinical and immunologic aspects of allergen-specific immunotherapy in patients with seasonal allergic rhinitis and/or allergic asthma. *J Allergy Clin Immunol* 1983: **72**: 323–4.

Chapter 9

NASAL POLYPS

A. B. Drake-Lee

INTRODUCTION

The word polyp was first used by Hippocrates to describe the nasal condition which had been described previously in India over one thousand five hundred years before Christ. It comes from the Greek words *poly-pous* and means many footed or feet. It is a descriptive term and does not imply a pathological mechanism. The term is most commonly used to describe simple, benign nasal polyps which are bilateral and arise from the ethmoid sinuses. When the term was first introduced it was used to describe all polypoid lesions encountered in the nose and therefore included neoplasms which are rare. Simple, mucous polyps were considered to be neoplastic conditions by some authors until well into the nineteenth century. Billroth described their histological features but considered them neoplastic [1]. This is not his only contribution to ENT since he performed one of the first laryngectomies. Zuckerkandl realised that they were inflammatory in nature.

DEFINITION

This chapter will concentrate on simple nasal polyps and they are usually found in both sides of the nose. They can occur on one side but they must be removed and examined histologically to exclude neoplasms.

Polyps are the linings of the ethmoid sinuses that prolapse into the nose where they appear as pale structures in the nasal cavity. The turbinates too can undergo polypoidal changes and also block the nose. Polyps may arise from the maxillary sinus and usually descend into the post nasal space and are visible here with the post nasal space mirror, they are called antrochoanal polyps and are a different entity.

Polyps have a constant histological character and so are usually considered as a single entity. The nose is only capable in acting in a number of ways and so the same histological picture may be produced by a number of different aetiologies. The same considerations hold true for a urethral stricture, for example. The aim of the ENT surgeon is to exclude rare known causes in some cases, from the majority of patients who have no obvious underlying cause.

Although, for reasons that become apparent later, most polyps are considered either due to allergy or infection, these premises are incorrect. Polyps are in general a disease of adults.

AETIOLOGY

Age

Polyps may arise in children but most of the children who are referred to the specialist have enlarged inferior turbinates that are mistaken for polyps. When they arise in children the age of onset is important. The ethmoid sinuses are not well enough developed before the age of two years for polyps to arise from here. If polyps are encountered then a defect of the anterior cranial floor should be suspected and the child have a computerised tomogram of the area performed. Primary biopsy is contraindicated. If they are seen after the age of two then they may be a presenting manifestation of cystic fibrosis [2]. Polyps usually arise in established cases and in some may be particularly recurrent. They may cause soft tissue expansion of the floor of the anterior cranial fossa and result in hypertelorism as the child grows.

Predisposing factors

Polyps occur in 8% of cases with cystic fibrosis [3] and they are associated with the respiratory rather than the gastrointestinal manifestations of the disease. This may help to explain the lack of increase in polyps in children now alive because of control of gastrointestinal symptoms in the first year of life and the better survival of those who present with meconium ileus.

While the deficit in cystic fibrosis is in the function of the exocrine glands, other abnormalities in the respiratory mucosa may result in polyp formation. Immotile cilial syndrome (Kartagener's syndrome) can eventually result in polyps because of stasis of mucus, as can hyperviscous mucus seen in Young's syndrome. These two are very rare causes of polyps in adults and often follow a long period of respiratory illness in childhood which should alert the clinician.

Benign simple polyps present mostly in adults and are rare before the age of 20. They occur for the first time in equal numbers of patients for each decade up to 60, after which they are encountered more rarely.

Incidence

The true incidence of polyps is difficult to determine but can be inferred from the incidence of late onset asthma. The numbers of patients with some degree of late onset asthma is about one per 100 and about one third of these patients have nasal polyps. Equally, about one third of patients with nasal polyps have some evidence of bronchospasm. It would appear that between one and 20 per 1000 of the adult population have nasal polyps at some time in their lives. This would fit in with the general incidence of nasal disease in the UK. Allergic rhinitis occurs in about 10% of the population and non-allergic rhinitis occurs in a further 5%. A proportion of the latter have nasal polyps.

Sex

A strong male predominance is found both in children with cystic fibrosis and adults who have nasal polyps. Figures vary from series to series but the ratio is between two and four to one. This is not found in patients who have asthma in addition to polyps where the incidence is the same [5]. This argues for a different group of patients who have asthma in addition to polyps as opposed to simple nasal polyps alone.

Racial groups

All racial groups have nasal polyps and as yet there are no comparable studies between the four major groups. Most of the published research work has dealt with people of European extraction and has been confirmed by workers in Japan.

143

Animal studies

Polyps are virtually confined to man, although there has been an occasional case in other primates, usually chimpanzees. Cats sometimes have a eustachian polyp and cows have granulation polyps of the nasal septum, but this is confined to cows of European extraction living in Australia. The differing development of the ethmoturbinal system in other animals may account for the species differences. This means that there are no animal models in which to study the disease processes and so work must be performed on human tissue.

Asthma and other respiratory diseases

The association between nasal polyps and other diseases, particularly asthma, has been widely accepted. Maloney and Collins [6] reviewed the literature and stated that between 20 and 40% of patients with polyps had some degree of bronchospasm. This is associated with late onset asthma rather than patients who develop asthma in childhood. The number of children with asthma is rising but around 5% have some evidence of asthma during childhood. The incidence of childhood asthma in cases of nasal polyps is 3.5% [5]. While the aetiology of asthma is extensively debated, cases developing asthma during childhood have a strong allergic bias.

Other diseases, such as cystic fibrosis, immotile cilial syndrome and Young's syndrome which result in an unstable respiratory mucosa, may result in the development of nasal polyps.

Aspirin hypersensitivity

There is a well recognised triad of asthma, aspirin hypersensitivity and nasal polyps. It occurs in up to 8% of patients who present with this condition. The mechanism is uncertain but it is not an allergic reaction and both prostaglandins [7] and leukotrienes [8] have been implicated in the production of the oedema. This is presumably mediated via mast cell degranulation.

Allergy

Allergy has, for some time, been considered to predispose to polyp

Table 1: The incidence of allergic diseases in nasal polyps

	Polyp patients	Normal population
Hayfever	10%	10%
Childhood asthma	5%	5%
Eczema	11%	3%
Penicillin allergy	7%	<15%
Positive skin tests	25%	20-25%
	Non allergic diseases	
Late onset asthma	>25%	3%
Apririn intolerance	8%	0.1%

formation but it is the result of a loose association of features. Histologically over 90% of polyps have a tissue eosinophilia, over 20% have asthma and many of the patients have a prodromal period of rhinitis with blockage, running and sneezing. The term ''allergy'' has been used in a number of ways but now is defined as a reaction of a known allergen with an allergen specific immunoglobulin (most commonly IgE) which is situated on a mast cell. Certain clinical conditions are known to be mediated by these reactions such as seasonal allergic rhinitis and perennial rhinitis caused by dust mite sensitivity. Several authors have felt that allergic diseases are no more common in polyp patients than in the normal population [5, 9]. Table 1 shows the incidence of allergic diseases in polyp patients compared with literature controls. Hay fever, childhood asthma, aspirin hypersensitivity (which may be mediated by IgE) and multiple positive skin tests are no more common than expected. The presence of allergy would appear to be coincidental and the presence of an allergic disease in patients is not associated with a more severe recurrence pattern.

Sinusitis

Virtually every patient with nasal polyps has extensive radiological changes in the sinuses which is not confined to the ethmoids from where most polyps arise, so that all patients have sinusitis. Unfortunately, sinusitis does not mean infected sinusitis as is commonly implied. Confusion comes from misunderstanding of the literature where two types of sinusitis are recognised, true infective sinusitis and hyperplastic sinusitis.

Purulent sinusitis results from infection, usually by bacteria, that may become chronic. Inflammation responds to appropriate treatment with antimicrobial chemotherapy and surgical treatment if necessary. The incidence of chronic sinusitis has decreased dramatically over the last fifty years and in this respect is like mastoiditis. Nasal polyps do not seem to have become any less frequent.

The mucosa taken from the sinuses of patients who have extensive surgery shows the same morphological features as the mucosa of the bronchi of equivalent patients dying in status asthmaticus. Hyperplastic sinusitis is associated with mucus hypersecretion and when the ostium of a sinus is blocked then secretions remain in the sinus. These may then become colonised and bacterial sinusitis ensues. The commonest organism cultured from the maxillary sinus is a non-capsulated *Haemophilus influenzae,* but well over 40% of the washouts have no return and half or more of these grow no organism [10]. A further study compared the radiographic features with washout findings and the presence of pus cells and found that out of 104 washouts, pus cells and organisms were found in only 16 [11]. The role of *H. influenzae* appears to be the same as in cases of chronic bronchitis.

A further indirect argument is the dramatic response of about half the cases to glucocorticosteroids. If the process were primarily infective then an exacerbation of the condition should occur, and even in those cases who do not respond there is no exacerbation of symptoms.

HISTOLOGY

The histological features of polyp tissue, sinus mucosa and the lining of the bronchii from patients dying in status asthmaticus are the same. Respiratory epithelium lies on a thickened basement membrane which covers a grossly oedamatous submucosa. The oedematous nature of the stroma has been well demonstrated histologically by Taylor [12]. If there has been repeated trauma to the polyp then the epithelium may undergo squamous metaplasia. The submucosa contains few vessels, which are mainly capillaries, and the cellular infiltrate is mainly plasma cells, small lymphocytes and macrophages, and (the most striking feature which is present in over 90% of polyps) an eosinophilia. The eosinophilia varies from polyp to polyp and from one part of a polyp to another. There is little nervous tissue. Some of the cells may show atypia in the stroma [13].

Mast cells

Although there is debate on the subgrouping of mast cells in animals, there does not appear to be any obvious distinct subgroups in man, more a spectrum of cells which have metachromatic granules at light microscopy and electron dense granules ultrastructurally. Ultrastructural studies have shown that mast cells in polyps are degranulated [14, 15]. The degranulation would give rise to the eosinophilia, and the presence of inflammatory mediators would account for the oedema.

Polyp oedema

The polyp oedema is easy to collect and this has been done in several studies, the first of which was reported by Berdal [16]. Serum may also be collected and levels of compounds compared in both samples from the same patient. The fluid is mainly oedema since all the plasma proteins may be demonstrated and are present in lower amounts than in serum. All the immunoglobulins are present but IgA and IgE are produced locally in greater amounts than can be accounted for by diffusion alone. Vasoactive compounds are found in mast cell degranulation, including histamine, prostaglandins and the leukotrienes. Histamine levels are, on average, several hundred times the serum levels [17]. These come from the mast cells that are degranulated and are well above the levels that have been encountered in nasal secretions. Local inflammatory reactions occur throughout the nose but the anatomical development of the ethmoids facilitates persistent oedema since the blood supply is far less well developed in the sinuses. The process is dynamic so that polyps may vary in size.

It has not been possible to show that mast cell reactions in polyps are either mediated by allergic reactions or are complement dependent.

SYMPTOMS AND SIGNS

Symptoms

Almost all patients have nasal obstruction to some degree. This is frequently bilateral although it is not always equal in severity.

Sometimes the obstruction is felt to be valve-like so that it varies on position. Sneezing and anterior rhinorrhoea are present in about half the patients and are frequently found together. A similar proportion of patients complain about loss of the senses of smell and taste. The grossly congested mucosa may produce excess mucus and the patient complains of a post nasal drip. If the material is infected then the mucus may become green; however, an eosinophilia may colour the mucus a yellowy green. Pain around the face is present occasionally but patients complain more frequently about pressure in the nose and face. Epistaxis is uncommon and suggests a more sinister condition.

Signs

Patients talk with a hyponasal voice and are often asked if they have a cold. If the polyps are severe then they can prolapse out of the nose but they are usually seen inside the nares where they appear as pale semitranslucent masses in the nasal cavity. If they are injected or the examiner cannot determine whether the structure is a polyp then it can be probed lightly. Polyps are relatively insensitive because they have a poor nerve supply.

If polyps are present before the facial bones fuse, as in children with cystic fibrosis, then the resulting pressure in the ethmoids will force the growing skull apart and produce hypertelorism. Polyps rarely produce bone erosion but it may be present following surgery and if the patient develops a mucocoele. The latter are very rare in polyp patients and usually arise following previous surgery.

Investigations

There are no diagnostic investigations in patients with nasal polyps. Radiology of the sinuses shows involvement of the sinuses to some degree in virtually every patient. This is contrasted with patients with allergic rhinitis where the sinuses are usually clear or only very minor changes are seen. Radiology has a much greater role in patients with a neoplasm who present with a unilateral nasal polyp. Surgeons who use the nasendoscope for resecting polyps advocate computerised scanning prior to surgery.

TREATMENT

Unfortunately much of the earlier work on nasal polyps was anecdotal, particularly regarding the need for surgery and its efficacy in preventing recurrence. Some authors felt that surgery caused asthma whereas they are both manifestations of the same pathology in the respiratory mucosa. If surgery does have any effect then it tends to improve the asthma [8]. This is logical since the nose resumes its normal physiological function and warms and humidifies the inspired air, preventing cold air entering the lungs and inducing bronchospasm in hyperreactive individuals.

Medical treatment prior to surgery

As mentioned earlier in the chapter, about half the cases respond to corticosteroids. Although polyps regress when corticosteroids are given orally, because of the risk of side effects when corticosteroids are administered by this route, they are usually given intranasally. It is worth trying corticosteroids on all patients since their use will prevent surgery in up to half of them. Betamethasone drops, two each side twice a day with retention should be tried, or an aqueous spray such as beclomethasone or flunisolide two puffs each side twice a day [18, 19]. All should be given for a trial period of a month. If the polyps do not respond, then they may be removed surgically.

Surgical treatment

There are many different views on the surgical treatment required for nasal polyps. The attitude to surgery is coloured by those patients who have severe recurrences. Many patients who have occasional recurrences, perhaps every 10 years, may be treated very effectively by simple polypectomy.

Unfortunately no trials have ever been performed on patients who have radical surgery despite the enthusiasm of some authors [20]. More recently intranasal ethmoidectomy by endoscopic resection has become popular on the continent of Europe and in some centres in the United States of America. The philosophy here is that ethmoidectomy will eradicate the disease and prevent recurrence but as yet no trial results have been published and the author knows of none in progress.

Intranasal ethmoidectomy is associated with orbital complications such as herniation of orbital fat, medial rectus palsy and, in severest cases, blindness. It also renders the middle turbinate unstable during surgery and it may thus be removed inadvertently. The loss of the middle turbinate makes subsequent surgery difficult since one of the main landmarks for intranasal surgery has gone. External ethmoidectomy is associated with periorbital scarring but does allow direct vision of the orbit. It would seem that in the absence of any data to support more extensive surgery, simple removal is the desired treatment.

Recurrence

This is not a complication of surgery but a problem in the management of some cases of nasal polyps. There is no way a surgeon can know beforehand which cases will recur, but an earlier age of onset is associated with more severe recurrence, as is the presence of asthma and aspirin hypersensitivity. These last two suggest a more aggressive respiratory mucosal disease.

Post operative therapy

The place of post-operative corticosteroids has yet to be determined but evidence suggests that long-term post-operative treatment reduces the severity of recurrence [21, 22]. Not all patients require therapy. Those with polyps who present for the first time and those with several years between recurrences do not necessarily require treatment. Patients who have rhinitis should be treated to control symptoms. Both beclomethasone and flunisolide or other fluorinated corticosteroid nasal sprays may be used.

Diets

Since there is a link between aspirin and the natural salicylates and tartrazine dyes, it is worth trying patients on a diet free from these compounds. It is difficult to perform controlled trials but about half the patients with aspirin hypersensitivity say that they felt better with fewer nasal symptoms. These diets do no harm and many patients would like to do something to help themselves.

CONCLUSIONS

Polyps are a multifactorial disease which affect the nasal lining and sinus mucosa and in about a third of the patients are associated with asthma. Polyps may occur in other respiratory diseases such as cystic fibrosis and immotile cilial syndrome. Allergy does not predispose to polyp formation but mast cell reactions appear to be important and may explain why corticosteroids are effective in controlling some cases and helping to prevent recurrence in others. Simple polypectomy is the treatment of choice in those cases requiring surgery.

REFERENCES

1. Vancil M. Histochemical studies on nasal polyps. *J Laryngol Otol* 1963; **77**: 326-41.
2. Lurie H. Cystic fibrosis of the pancreas and the nasal mucosa. *Ann Otol Rhinol Laryngol* 1959; **68**: 478.
3. Schwachman H, Kulcyzchi I, Mueller H, Flake C. Nasal polyposis in patients with cystic fibrosis. *Paediatrics* 1962; **30**: 389-401.
4. Drake-Lee A, Barker T, Thurley K. Nasal polyps II. Fine structure of mast cells. *J Laryngol Otol* 1984; **98**: 285-92.
5. Drake-Lee A, Lowe D, Swanston A, Grace A. Clinical profile and recurrence of nasal polyps. *J Laryngol Otol* 1984; **98**: 783-93.
6. Maloney J, Collins J. Nasal polyps and bronchial asthma. *Br J Dis Chest* 1977; **71**: 1-6.
7. Sczeklik A, Gryglewski R, Czerniawske-Mysik G. Relationship of inhibition of prostaglandin biosynthesis by analgesics to asthma attacks in aspirin sensitive patients. *Br Med J* 1975; **1**: 67-9.
8. Maloney J. Nasal polyps, nasal polypectomy, asthma and aspirin sensitivity. *J Laryngol Otol* 1977; **91**: 837-46.
9. Settipane G, Chafee F. Nasal polyps in asthma and rhinitis. *J Allergy Clin Immunol* 1977; **58**: 17-21.
10. Majumdar B, Bull P. The incidence of maxillary sinusitis in nasal polyps. *J Laryngol Otol* 1982; **96**: 927-42.
11. Dawes P, Bates G, Watson D, Lewis D, Lowe D, Drake-Lee A. The role of bacterial infection of the maxillary sinus in nasal polyps. *Clin Otolaryngol*. In press.
12. Taylor M. Histochemical studies on nasal polyps. *J Laryngol Otol* 1963; **77**: 326-41.
13. Freedman I, Osborne D, eds. Miscellaneous granulomas and nasal polyps. In: *Pathology of granulomas and neoplasms of the nose and paranasal sinuses*. Edinburgh: Churchill Livingstone, 1982; 28-35.
14. Cauna N, Hindover K, Manzethi G, Swanson E. Fine structure of nasal polyps. *Ann Otol Rhinol Laryngol* 1972; **81**: 41-58.
15. Drake-Lee A, Barker T, Thurley K. Nasal polyps II. Fine structure of mast cells. *J Laryngol Otol* 1984; **98**: 285-92.
16. Berdal P. Serological examination of nasal polyp fluid. *Acta Otolaryngologica* 1954; Suppl 115.
17. Drake-Lee A, McLaughlan P. Clinical symptoms, free histamine and IgE in patients with nasal polyps. *Int Arch Allergy Appl Immunol* 1982; **69**: 268-71.
18. Charlton R, MacKay I, Wilson R, Cole P. Double blind placebo controlled trial of beclomethasone nose drops for nasal polyps. *Br Med J* 1985; **2**: 788-9.

19. Dingsor G, Kramer J, Olsholt R, Sonderstrom J. Flunisolide nasal spray 0.025% in the prophylactic treatment of nasal polyposis after polypectomy. *Rhinology* 1985; **23**: 49-53.
20. Hughes R. The role of radical surgery in the treatment of nasal polyps. *J Laryngol Otol* 1973; **87**: 117-22.
21. Mygind N, Pedersen C, Prytz S, Sorensen H. Treatment of nasal polyps with intranasal beclomethasone dipropionate aerosol. *Clin Allergy* 1975; **5**: 159-64.
22. Dueschl L, Dretner B. Nasal polyps treated by beclomethasone nasal aerosol. *Rhinology* 1977; **15**: 17-23.

Chapter 10

SINUSITIS: DIAGNOSIS AND TREATMENT

Valerie J. Lund

INTRODUCTION

Sinusitis has been defined as an inflammation of the mucous membrane of the paranasal sinuses resulting from inadequate drainage usually secondary to physical obstruction, infection or allergy [1]. However, it is a broad term covering a condition which affects one or more of the sinuses in both children and adults, and varies in degree from acute to chronic. The sinuses cannot be regarded in isolation and the condition should really be considered as rhinosinusitis. Whilst it is usually possible to diagnose acute sinusitis, it is much more difficult to interpret the transition which occurs through acute recurrent attacks and the subacute state to the chronic situation. This in turn must be distinguished from a number of other conditions producing some similar symptoms and consideration given to possible contributory factors.

The maxillary sinus is most often affected acutely, though any or all of the other sinuses may be involved at the same time and this is particularly the case as chronicity develops. Pathologically acute sinusitis is characterised by hyperaemia, haemorrhage and submucosal oedema with polymorphonuclear infiltration [2]. In uncomplicated cases the periosteum and bone remain intact but rapid erosion can be seen in fulminating disease. The subacute situation is said to demonstrate a proliferation of young connective tissue but it is difficult to establish at what point it becomes chronic with irreversible change to mucus-secreting elements, squamous metaplasia of ciliated epithelium, necrosis and periosteal and bone reaction leading to sclerosis. The distinction between these definitions has important implications on the likely efficacy of our therapeutic options.

DIAGNOSIS

History

A careful history will, as usual, give the best indication of the condition. Many patients attribute facial pain to "sinus" and it is important to distinguish this from other causes such as temporal arteritis, migraine, trigeminal neuralgia or pain of dental origin. Although the pain of acute sinusitis may be localised over the respective sinus as in maxillary, ethmoidal or frontal infection or be retro-orbital or occipital in the case of the sphenoid, more often several areas may be affected, particularly as more than one sinus is often involved. Classically it is described as a pressure sensation, increased by bending down or straining. In chronic sinusitis the distribution of pain is more diffuse and the degree dependent on individual variation.

In acute sinusitis, the symptoms usually develop following an upper respiratory tract infection. Occasionally other events may precede the attack, such as severe facial trauma with secondary infection or haemorrhage. Barotrauma and diving have also been cited as causative factors though they are only likely to be a problem in the presence of an existing "cold".

When acute infection appears to occur spontaneously, especially when recurrent, the possibility of other underlying conditions should be considered and will require further investigation (*vide infra*). Primary ciliary and mucus abnormalities most frequently present with lower respiratory tract infections or infertility though it may be that the less serious upper respiratory tract symptoms have been overlooked. Patients with immune deficiency (congenital or acquired), may also present with other infective manifestations but it is not unusual for the upper respiratory tract to be one of the earliest areas affected.

In both acute and chronic situations, nasal obstruction is experienced mainly due to oedema of the mucosa though it may be exacerbated by contributory anatomical abnormalities. Discharge, both in anterior rhinorrhoea and postnasal catarrh, can lead to confusion in interpretation. If there is an underlying rhinitis (allergic or non-allergic) a watery rhinorrhoea may be present. However, in a straightforward acute bacterial sinusitis, the ostium of that sinus is generally obstructed and there may be no obvious flow into the nasal cavity. Once the ostium reopens, the purulent secretion is discharged, as the "abscess" resolves. In contradistinction, in the chronic situation, patients complain bitterly of a persistent mucopurulent discharge flowing into the postnasal space, causing coughing, voice changes and retching, particularly in the morning. The persistence of the postnasal discharge following an acute episode marks the transition to chronicity, and is evidence of the pathophysiological changes occurring in the mucus-secreting elements and ciliary mechanisms. Conversely, it should be remembered that not all purulent secretions result from infection.

Complaints of swelling or tenderness over the sinuses do occur in acute sinusitis but should alert one in the case of the maxilla to a dental origin for the infection or to the possibility of an imminent complication. The constitutional effects of sinusitis may also vary though most patients feel unwell and have a pyrexia in the acute stage.

Examination

An adequate examination of the ears, nose and throat is possible without the aid of specialist instrumentation, using an auroscope for the ears and nose, and tongue depressors for the mouth. Other sources of infection such as the tonsils may be demonstrated and particular attention should be paid to the dentition which should be tapped and palpated as it is estimated that 10% of all cases of maxillary sinusitis are dental in origin [3].

Anterior rhinoscopy may reveal an obvious anatomical abnormality such as a deviated septum, hypertrophied inferior turbinates, or a foreign body, polyps or even something more sinister. Pus may be seen in the middle meatus, or running down the posterior pharyngeal wall. However, often no abnormality other than some reddening and oedema of the nasal mucosa may be evident.

Other signs of predisposing conditions may be seen: the conjunctivitis of seasonal allergy, respiratory evidence of asthma or bronchiectasis, serous otitis media in disturbances of mucocilary clearance or the ENT manifestations of AIDS. These latter include a granular change in the nasal mucosa similar to that found in sarcoid, oral candida, otitis externa, cervical lymphadenopathy and Kaposi's sarcoma.

At this point the clinician may institute treatment without resort to further investigation. Clearly many of the following techniques are applicable only after specialist referral and indeed in some cases only available to a small number of ENT surgeons with an interest in rhinology. However, whilst the majority of patients can be managed primarily, it is worth remembering the other possible lines of investigation which may be of importance in a minority of intractable cases.

Radiology

Three plain sinus X-ray views are performed routinely: occipito-mental, occipito-frontal and lateral. In acute sinusitis, particularly of the maxilla, oedematous swelling of the mucosa results in a peripheral opaque rim parallel to the walls of the sinus. This is said to contrast with that occurring in allergic sinusitis in which polypoid change occurs with a convex inner border. The situation, however, is rarely so straightforward [4]. More usually gross mucosal thickening and/or exudation of fluid into the obstructed cavity results in varying degrees of opacification. To determine the presence of a fluid level, a tilt view should be performed but after allowing a few minutes to elapse so thick secretion can assume the new level (Fig. 1).

CT and MRI will obviously show fluid and oedematous mucosa (especially on T2 weighted spin echo sequences of MRI) but these techniques are rarely indicated except when excluding neoplasia, demonstrating complications such as osteomyelitis, frontal lobe abscesses or orbital cellulitis and when contemplating surgery on the fronto-ethmoidal complex.

In the chronic situation mucosal thickening predominates but sclerosis of adjacent bony walls may be seen associated with long-standing proliferative osteitis, particularly in the frontal bone. Bearing in mind other contributory conditions such as sarcoid, a chest X-ray is mandatory in recurrent or chronic cases.

Ultrasound

The technique of distinguishing solid, fluid and air by sound waves has achieved little popularity in Great Britain. However, considerable experience and success have been claimed in other parts of Europe suggesting good radiological correlation [5].

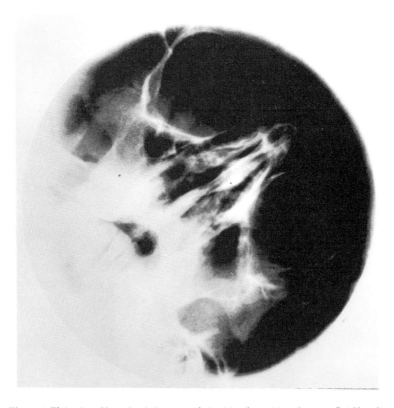

Figure 1: Plain sinus X-ray (occipito-mental view) in tilt position showing fluid level in right maxillary sinus and opacification on left.

Sinus puncture, bacteriology and endoscopy

In the past, puncture of the maxillary antrum and lavage constituted the mainstay of therapy in the pre-antibiotic era and subsequently when medication failed. This has been superceded, where facilities are available, by fibreoptic endoscopy which allows diagnosis (both histological and bacteriological) and treatment. The ethmoids are not amenable to such examination and it is safer to use external trephination of the frontal sinus than to try and navigate the frontonasal duct, but the rigid Hopkins rod (2.7 or 4 mm diameter, 0', 30' or 70') allows a thorough examination of the nasal cavity after adequate local anaesthesia and visualisation of the ostia of the respective sinuses revealing the origin of purulent secretion and causes of obstruction (Fig. 2).

157

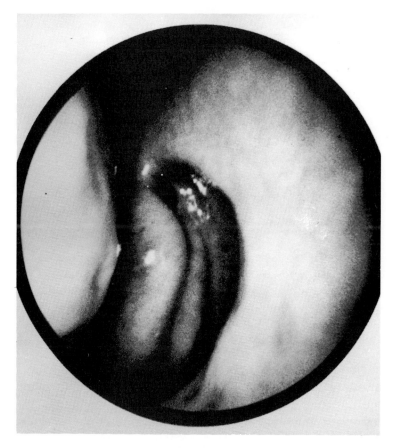

Figure 2: Photograph of view of middle meatus through 4 mm O'Hopkins rod, showing accessory maxillary sinus ostium.

Entry of the maxillary sinus is most safely encompassed via the inferior meatus or canine fossa and can be performed under local or general anaesthesia. The inferior route is perhaps technically easier but does not afford such a good view of the ostial area even with 70′ scopes. Having entered the sinus, secretion can be aspirated directly, biopsies taken for culture and histology, lavage performed and small intrasinus manipulations performed such as marsupialisation of cysts.

The vexed question of microbiology in this condition deserves special consideration. We usually think of sinusitis as being bacterial. However, it is possible for sterile secretions to accumulate in any one of the sinuses in response to allergic and non-allergic

Table 1: Microbiology of acute sinusitis

Streptococcus pneumoniae	31–44%
Haemophilus influenzae	21–35%
Klebsiella spp	

a
b } Haemolytic streptococcus
c

Staphylococcus aureus
Pseudomonas spp
Branhamella catarrhalis
Enterobacteria spp
Anaerobes—fusobacteria
 —anaerobic streptococci
 —*Bacteroides* spp
Viruses—rhinovirus
 —parainfluenza
 —influenza

rhinosinusitis. When sinusitis follows an upper respiratory tract infection, the initiating pathogen is viral and this may account for the high number of negative bacterial cultures from even carefully collected sinus aspirates. Rhinovirus, parainfluenza and influenza have all been cultured from acute maxillary sinusitis [6,7].

Once bacterial infection supervenes a number of common pathogens are found, the commonest of these being *Streptococcus pneumoniae* and *Haemophilus influenzae* which account for 50% of proven infections (Table 1) [8]. However, as can be seen, a wide range of organisms may be found including anaerobes. The incidence of anaerobes increases in chronic sinusitis where they may constitute up to 30% of infections [8–10]. *H. influenzae* and *Strep. pneumoniae* again are found but there is also a much higher incidence of *Staphylococcus aureus*. The increased prevalence of anaerobes may reflect the low oxygen concentration and impaired mucosal blood flow resulting from a chronically obstructed sinus. Recently interest has grown in *Branhamella catarrhalis* (*Neisseria catarrhalis*) which may act as a primary pathogen or facilitate the pathogenicity of other organisms. The emergence of beta-lactam producing strains of bacteria may also influence medical management of the condition [11].

It is important to note that whilst the nasal cavity and paranasal sinuses are sterile, many of these potentially pathogenic organisms are found colonising the nasal vestibule and nasopharynx of normal subjects [12]. It may be that the primary viral infection disrupts mucociliary mechanisms allowing secondary bacterial invasion by commensals. However, it is also clear from a number of studies that the correlation between nasal swabs and antral contents obtained by sterile puncture is poor and therefore cannot be relied on to aid therapeutic choice [13].

Rarely fungal infections can occur in the sinuses. These can take an aggressive fulminant course in the immunocompromised or debilitated host [14] but can also produce an "allergic" reaction with minimal soft tissue invasion in normal subjects who have usually spent time abroad [15]. The commonest mycotic agents are *Aspergillus flavus* and *A. fumigatus* but *A. conidiobolus* and *A. mucormycosis* can also occur.

As previously mentioned "purulent" secretion need not necessarily reflect a pathogen and may occur due to an abundance of eosinophils in the secretion which can be revealed by a nasal smear.

The following investigations have been discussed in earlier chapters but should be mentioned for completeness.

Skin prick tests

Allergy alone may lead to a sterile sinusitis and polypoid mucosal change. This in turn may result in ostial obstruction and stasis with secondary bacterial infection. Skin prick tests, including negative and positive controls should be performed on all patients but remembering diminishing responsiveness with age and the effect of concomitant medication. The results compare favourably both in reliability and cost with the more sophisticated RAST tests.

Blood tests

A full blood count, ESR, urea, electrolytes and liver function tests may reveal an underlying contributory medical condition. In addition an assessment of immune status is most important as it becomes increasingly realised that a proportion of patients with recurrent upper respiratory tract infections are immunodeficient [18]. Routine serum immunoglobulin levels may show a deficiency of one class but even in the presence of normal values, subclass analysis may demonstrate a specific deficiency. Similarly a small group of patients lack certain immunoglobulin in the saliva and nasal mucus though clearly these investigations are only available at a limited number of laboratories after specialist referral. Of more immediate concern is the possibility of AIDS which can present with an apparently simple acute sinusitis.

Nasomucociliary clearance (Fig. 3)

Complex patterns of mucus drainage operate within the nose and sinuses carrying it in predetermined paths to the natural ostia. Primary abnormalities of the cilia as in primary cilial dyskinesia and primary abnormalities of mucus as in Young's syndrome are rare but secondary abnormalities are very common and recent work has shown the effect of bacterial infection in slowing, stopping and destroying the ciliated mucosa of the respiratory tract [19]. A simple test for the evaluation of this mechanism exists and consists of placing a small piece of saccharine on the anterior end of the inferior turbinate [20]. Normally a sweet taste appears in the mouth within 30 minutes, evidence of the change in nasal mucus blanket twice an hour. Cases in excess of this, assuming the test has been carried out correctly, can be further assessed by a ciliary brushing and the ciliary beat frequency measured directly using a special microscope with photometric cell [21].

TREATMENT

The investigations discussed are not applicable to all patients but may define a small group with persistent problems who will require specific replacement and long-term antibiotics and can be spared more radical surgical treatment which is unlikely to provide long-term benefit. In the remaining majority our management options will be medical, surgical or a combination of both.

Medical

In the presence of obvious infection, a broad spectrum antibiotic such as amoxycillin, ampicillin or cotrimoxazole is indicated. If there is minimal clinical response the possibility of beta-lactam activity and anaerobic infection should be considered, suggesting the use of cefuroxime axetil, amoxicillin/clavulanate or the addition of metronidazole. It has been argued that no antibiotic therapy is indicated at all, particularly in the acute situation which may be viral,

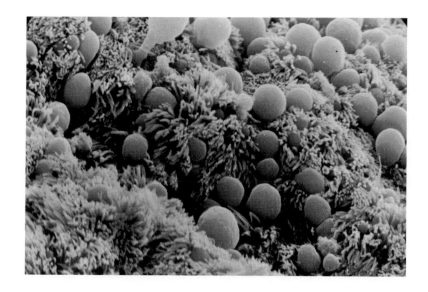

Figure 3: Electron micrograph (magnification × 2097) showing ciliated columnar epithelium of nasal cavity with mucus extruding from goblet cells.

as the majority of cases will resolve spontaneously. However, once bacterial infection has become established, it would seem that the general morbidity of the patient and the incidence of complications which are rarely seen nowadays, are significantly diminished by therapeutic intervention. It is also possible that prompt medical treatment may ultimately diminish the incidence of irreversible damage to mucociliary mechanisms, resulting in chronic sinusitis. The pain will require an appropriate analgesic and to establish drainage it is worth considering a short course of decongestant drops.

In the chronic situation, topical intranasal steroids, can be of considerable benefit, in particular betamethasone administered in the head down and forwards position which seem effective in diminishing mucopurulent catarrh [22]. It is difficult to evaluate accurately the effects of the many available sympathomimetic decongestants and antihistamines though some patients find them of help. Sometimes a long course of broad spectrum antibiotic may also be of benefit.

Surgical (Table 2)

If medical treatment prescribed by the GP or ENT surgeon fails we have to decide what surgical procedure is most appropriate [23]. As already mentioned, irrigation of the sinus is a useful diagnostic and therapeutic procedure which can be a simple "antral washout" or employ sinoscopy under local or general anaesthesia.

Certainly the old regime of one washout every week for six weeks would be unacceptable to most patients and their ENT surgeons these days and the majority would proceed to a more definitive drainage procedure after failure to respond to a couple of washouts. Catheterisation of the maxillary sinus has been used but requires a well-motivated patient to perform their own frequent lavage.

Whilst the maxillary sinus is usually regarded as the commonest site of infection, the sinuses should be regarded as an integral unit and recent research has emphasised the role of the antro-ethmoidal complex leading to a resurgence of interest in surgery on the middle meatus and ethmoids [24,25]. Patients with limited disease in this region are amenable to such "functional" surgery but unfortunately many patients have extensive and generalised disease. Traditionally there has been a concentration on the maxillary sinus and inferior

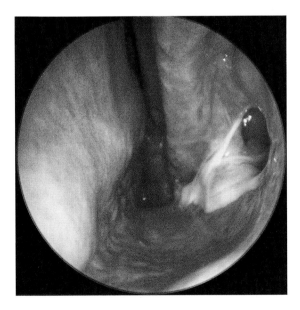

Figure 4: Photograph of view of inferior meatal antrostomy with pus running out.

Table 2: Surgical treatment in sinusitis

Maxillary sinus
  Conservative
    antral washout
    intranasal antrostomy
  Radical
    Caldwell-Luc
Fronto-ethmoidal complex
  Conservative
    trephination of frontal
    intranasal ethmoidectomy
    transantral ethmoidectomy
  Radical
    external fronto-ethmoidectomy
    osteoplastic flap

---

meatal antrostomy is commonly offered in combination with correction of any contributing anatomical abnormality such as hypertrophied inferior turbinates or a deviated nasal septum.

Enlarging the natural ostium of the maxillary sinus in the middle meatus can be performed but was not popular in the past due to the potential for damaging the optic nerve. However, better visualisation with fibre-optic illumination may result in this operation being performed more often in the future.

The rationale for an antrostomy is one of drainage of mucopurulent secretion and aeration of the sinus [26]. Infection disturbs the normal muco-ciliary patterns due to cilial damage and increased abnormal mucus production. However, performing an inferior meatal antrostomy in isolation ignores the relationship of the antrum and ethmoids and also assumes reversible mucosal change. Unfortunately when these changes become irreversible, the inferior meatal antrostomy may drain too well, principally by gravity, leading to an increase in mucopurulent catarrh (Fig. 4).

The patient may then be offered a Caldwell-Luc procedure which aims to cure by stripping out all the chronically infected maxillary sinus mucosa which in turn is replaced by fibrous tissue. This is equally unphysiological but may reduce post-nasal discharge. Ethmoidal disease can be exenterated intranasally and more safely than in the past using fibreoptic illumination or by using a transantral approach in combination with the Caldwell-Luc but for extensive disease an external approach is preferred by most surgeons in Great Britain.

Acute frontal or ethmoidal sinusitis is less commonly seen but must be recognised as the complications can be severe and rapid in

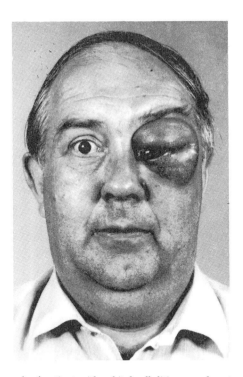

Figure 5: Photograph of patient with orbital cellulitis secondary to acute sinusitis.

onset. The frontal sinus is not present at birth and only develops fully in late teens, so acute infections occur from early adulthood onwards However, children can present with very dramatic ethmoiditis 24–48 hours into an upper respiratory tract infection. In both cases significant orbital cellulitis may be present which constitutes an emergency. It is often difficult to recognise the source of infection and many patients are referred to ENT surgeons from ophthamologists. Unless medical or surgical decompression of the orbit is instituted, vision may be permanently lost. Parenteral antibiotics should be instituted immediately (broad spectrum and anti-anaerobic combination such as cefuroxime and metronidazole) and vision carefully and regularly assessed (Fig. 5).

Colour vision is often affected first and any deterioration requires rapid surgical intervention. The frontal sinus can be trephined directly through a small skin incision under the medial brow but it is preferable to perform a formal external fronto-ethmoidectomy which establishes drainage of the cavity immediately as otherwise it is often required as a secondary procedure.

In the chronic situation all diseased mucosa can be removed by this approach, including the sphenoid sinus, and a permanent drainage channel established using a silastic tube or stent. This should be left *in situ* for as long as can be tolerated (preferably five months) and is removed in the outpatient department. Many more extensive procedures have been described for chronic frontal sinusitis ranging from the osteoplastic flap to total sinusectomy but are rarely if ever indicated and are cosmetically less satisfactory than the external fronto-ethmoidectomy operation. Conversely, it may be possible to improve frontal sinus drainage using intranasal endoscopic techniques but this requires considerable experience and large long-term follow-up studies are not yet available.

Dealing with acute sinusitis is usually straightforward but at present techniques to determine the degree of damage which marks the transition of acute to chronic infection are only experimental. However, an awareness of the possible aetiological and predisposing factors is clearly important so that patients may be offered the most appropriate and expeditious treatment thereby pre-empting the difficult management problems of chronic disease.

REFERENCES

1. Goldman JL. Infectious rhinitis and sinusitis. In: Goldmann JL, ed. *The principles and practice of rhinology*. New York: Wiley, 1987; 249–54.
2. Van Cauwenberge PB. Sinusitis. In: Braude AI, ed. *Medical microbiology and infectious diseases*. Philadelphia: WB Saunders, 1982; 825–34.
3. Waldman RH. Sinusitis. In: Waldman RH, Kluge RM, eds. *Infectious diseases*. New York: Medical Examination Publishing Co., 1984; 138– 43.
4. Lloyd GAS. Inflammatory and allergic sinus diseases. In: *Diagnostic imaging of the nose and paranasal sinuses*. Berlin, Heidelberg: Springer-Verlag, 1988; 41–50.
5. Bockmann P, Andersson L, Holmer NG, Jannert M, Lorinc P. Ultrasonic versus radiologic investigation of the paranasal sinuses. *Rhinology* 1982; **20**: 111–19.
6. Evans FO Jr, Sydnor JB, Moore WEC, *et al*. Sinusitis of the maxillary antrum. *N Engl J Med* 1975; **293**: 735–9.
7. Hamory BH, Sande MA, Sydnor A, *et al*. Etiology and antimicrobial therapy of acute maxillary sinusitis. *J Infect Dis* 1979; **139**: 197–202.
8. Verschraegen G. Which germs do we find in sinusitis and why? *Acta Otorhinolaryngol Belg* 1983; **37**: 584–8.
9. Frederick KJ, Braude AI. Anaerobic infection of the paranasal sinuses. *N Engl J Med* 1974; **290**: 135–7.
10. Su W, Liu C, Hung SY, *et al*. Bacteriological study in chronic maxillary sinusitis. *Laryngoscope* 1983; **93**: 931–4.
11. Sydnor A, Gwaltney JM, Scheld WM. The etiology and antimicrobial treatment of acute maxillary sinusitis in adults. In: Phillips I, ed. *Issues in the treatment of upper respiratory tract infection*. London, International Congress and Symposium Series No. 130, Royal Society of Medicine Services 1988; 31–9.

12. Gwaltney JM, Hayden FG. The nose and infection. In: Proctor DF, Andersen IB, eds. *The nose*. Amsterdam: Elsevier, 1982; 399–422.
13. Axelsson A, Brorson JE. The correlation between bacteriological findings in the nose and maxillary sinus in acute maxillary sinusitis. *Laryngoscope* 1973; **83**: 2003–11.
14. Antoine GA, Gates RH, Park AO. Invasive aspergillosis in a patient with aplastic anaemia receiving amphotericin B. *Head Neck Surg* 1988; **10**: 199–203.
15. Waxman JE, Spector JG, Sale SR. Allergic aspergillus sinusitis and treatment of a new clinical entity. *Laryngoscope* 1987; **97**: 261–6.
16. Illum P, Jeppesen P, Langebaeck E. X-ray examination and sinoscopy in maxillary sinus disease. *Acta Otolaryngol* 1972; **74**: 287– 92.
17. Herberhold C. Endoscopy of the maxillary sinus. *J Maxillofac Surg* 1973; **1**: 125–8.
18. Cole PJ. Immunity deficiency states. In: Scadding JG, Cumming G, eds. *Scientific foundations of respiratory medicine*. London: Heinemann, 1981: 441.
19. Wilson R, Sykes DA, Currie D, Cole PJ. Beat frequency of cilia from sites of purulent infection. *Thorax* 1986; **41**: 453–8.
20. Andersen IB, Camner P, Jensen PL, Philipson K, Proctor DF. Nasal clearance in monozygotic twins. *Am Rev Resp Dis* 1974; **110**: 301–5.
21. Rutland J, Dewar A, Cox T, Cole P. Nasal brushing for the study of ciliary ultrastructure. *J Clin Path* 1982; **35**: 357–9.
22. Wilson R, Sykes DA, Chan KL, Cole PJ, Mackay IS. The effect of head position on the efficacy of topical treatment of chronic mucopurulent rhino-sinusitis. *Thorax* 1987; **42**: 631–2.
23. Lund-VJ. Surgical management of sinusitis. In: Mackay IS, Bull TR, eds. *Scott-Brown's Otolaryngology, Vol. 4. Rhinology*, London: Butterworths, 1987; 180–202.
24. Stammberger H. Endoscopic endonasal surgery—concepts in treatment of recurring rhinosinusitis. *Otolaryngol Head Neck Surg* 1986; **94**: 143–56.
25. Kennedy DW, Zinreich SJ, Johns ME. Functional endoscopic sinus surgery. In: Goldman JL, ed. *The principles and practice of rhinology*. New York: Wiley; 1987; 879–902.
26. Lund VJ. Inferior meatal antrostomy. *J Laryngol Otol* 1988; Suppl 15.

Chapter 11

TOPICAL MEDICAL MANAGEMENT OF ALLERGIC CONDITIONS OF THE NOSE
Part 1: TOPICAL MEDICAL TREATMENT (EXCLUDING INTRANASAL STEROIDS)

D. A. Wong and J. Dolovich

INTRODUCTION

Topical nasal therapy for rhinitis is as appropriate today as it was to the ancients centuries ago. The rationale that local application of a beneficial substance would avoid the potentially adverse systemic effects of that substance rings true now as it did then. The Talmud prescribes ''dung of white dog mixed with myrrh'' while the Hindus used ''pepper, mustard, oris root, and asafoetida'' [1] to clean the nasal passages. The systemic use of such remedies would undoubtedly have been less popular. Even today the disadvantages of systemic medication can be avoided by topical medication with its attendant low systemic exposure. with the elucidation of the mechanisms responsible for the pathogenesis of the allergic reactions, a succession of drugs have been found which are effective in allergic rhinitis. Initially vasoconstrictors were introduced. Subsequently antihistamines, anticholinergics, sodium cromo-glycate, and steroids have come to have a place in topical treatment. With the introduction of these medications, there is an increasing number of controlled studies on the therapy of nasal allergy. On the other hand, non-allergic rhinitis continues to be poorly studied.

METHOD OF TOPICAL APPLICATION

Successful topical nasal therapy requires the use of appropriate methods of application of the medication to the nasal mucosa. Despite the importance of this subject to the effectiveness of therapy, little is known about the distribution of medication applied intranasally especially in the presence of increased secretions.

There are four different methods now in use: nasal drops, plastic spray bottles, freon-propelled pressurised aerosol and metered pump spray bottles. The use of drops of medication is effective only if the medication is in an appropriate formulation to allow adequate volumes to be distributed throughout the nasal mucosa. That is, multiple drops of a lower concentration of medication would be undoubtedly more effective than the same total dose in one or two drops of concentrated fluid in achieving wide distribution over the entire area of mucosa. Two methods of installation have been advocated to improve distribution. One is the traditional head back method followed by positioning of the head to one side and then the other and then forward [2]. Another is the installation of the drops while the patient is in the kneeling position with the top of his head towards the floor and face close to his knees. After giving the drops, the position is held for two minutes before standing [3]. Patient compliance with these methods may be low, however, and sprays of different types have become popular.

The inexpensive plastic squeeze bottle nebuliser is common in non-prescription drugs but is far from the best alternative. Although there is fairly good distribution of the drug nasally, the dose applied is highly dependent on the pressure used on the bottle. Men have been shown to give larger doses than women using the same bottle [4]. Children may develop systemic side effects with vasoactive amines from large doses inadvertently administered by adults [2]. As a result they are contraindicated in children, especially infants. The development of freon-propelled pressurised aerosols as used in inhalers for lower airway disease, allows for precise dosage and fairly even distribution especially if two puffs are directed at a slightly different angle [4]. If not properly aimed in the sagittal plane, however, there is a tendency for the particles to embed themselves in the mucosa causing local irritation rather than spreading evenly. The use of a metered pump, now available for some medications, is probably the best choice. The mechanical pump delivers a precise volume of medication at low pressure avoiding the pitfalls of previous devices, allowing for ease of use and good distribution with little irritation.

In topical aerosol therapy of rhinitis, like asthma, many failures are likely due to a faulty method of application. For effective inhalant therapy, careful instruction and observation of the method used by the patient has been proven to be vital. The same is likely true with topical nasal therapy.

NON-PHARMACOLOGICAL TOPICAL THERAPY

Wetting agents have a long history of use in the treatment of rhinitis. The installation of saline alone has been shown to improve symptoms from baseline as well as improve the biopsy appearance [5]. Also, when compared with medicated phenylephrine nasal drops, saline was at least as effective [6]. There have been three suggested methods of administering saline [7]: 1) commercial buffered saline in various spraying devices to be used regularly or as needed, 2) the mixture of a quarter teaspoon salt and seven ounces of water, used with a bulb syringe wherein the solution is infused into one nostril then the other, with head held over the sink, to allow the saline to run out through the other nostril, and 3) more recently, the availability of an affordable fluid infusion device, a Water Pik, allows one to mix a saline solution (one teaspoon with 800 ml of water) and infuse the saline in a fashion similar to 2). These regimens may be useful to prepare the nasal mucosa in severe cases for the subsequent use of other topical medications. The long term effectiveness, side effects and compliance with these methods have not been tested.

The use of inhaled humidified warm air, however, has received two large short-term studies [8, 9]. In one study sham devices were included in a double blind fashion; there was significant improvement in symptoms in the actively treated group [8]. A device which provides warmed humidified air for 30 minutes two or three times within one day has been claimed to have a lasting effect as long as a month on nasal symptoms. This apparently harmless therapy could be of benefit to some patients. Further studies, including comparisons with other modes of therapy, are required.

The safety and cost of non-pharmacological therapy make its use attractive, alone, or in combination with other modes of therapy. Its precise place has yet to be defined.

VASOACTIVE AMINES

The Chinese discovered the use of several herbs containing ephedrine for the treatment of coryza more than 5000 years ago. Emperor Shen Nung in 2735 BC listed several ephedrine containing substances as well as toads' eyelids for nasal symptoms [10]. The modern use of vasoconstrictors began with the isolation of the alkaloid, ephedrine, from the Chinese herb Ma-Huang in 1887 [11]. This was followed by the discovery and synthesis of epinephrine [12]. Phenylephrine was studied by Barger and Dale in 1902 [13]. In 1941 the first of the imidazaline derivatives, napholine was discovered. Although the adverse affects of these drugs were starting to be noticed, wide advertising of their benefits without warning led Kully in 1945 to report that no class of drugs was more widely distributed and used than the vasoconstrictors [11]. They continue to be widely used, and unfortunately abused, today.

Sympathomimetics are classified into two groups depending on the action on alpha receptors, which causes vasoconstriction, or beta receptors, which leads to vasodilation. The use of vasoactive amines, initially the sympathomimetics adrenaline and ephedrine, and then the safer imidazaline derivatives is based on their ability to produce vasoconstriction, reducing blood flow in resistance vessels as well as the volume of the capacitance vessels such as the cavernous sinusoids thereby increasing the patency of the nasal passages, and also decrease secretions. Beta stimulation has a detrimental vasodilatation effect but there is also a beneficial stabilisation of mast cells. The imidazaline derivatives, oxymetazoline and xylometazoline, are primarily alpha agonists with long-lasting effects, and apparently less rebound phenomenon, making them safer [14]. Although they effectively relieve nasal congestion quickly, it is presently considered that they should not be used in the long term management of chronic rhinitis due to apparent local complications. They provide useful acute relief or prevention of nasal congestion in situations such as bacterial or viral nasal mucosal infections, symptoms of eustachian tube blockage associated with air travel, and severe congestion secondary to allergy where acute vasoconstriction allows for examination and administration of other nasal medication [15]. A reasonable plan is to restrict the use to three to five days; more prolonged treatment can lead to rhinitis medicamentosa.

Adverse local effects of the long term topical nasal use of alpha agonists have been known for many years. Fox initially sounded the alarm in 1931 but few took notice [15]. Many cases of chronic regular use, which has been referred to as ''addiction'', have since been seen [16, 17]. The pathogenesis is still uncertain but may include a rebound vasodilatation giving rise to nasal stuffiness. This effect may be secondary to mucosal ischaemia from the initial

172

vasoconstriction, a beta agonist action which outlasts the alpha agonist effect or possibly an alpha adrenergic agonist-induced down-regulation of corresponding adrenergic receptors. This rebound effect, particularly from the nonspecific sympathomimetics, sometimes leads to greater congestion than when the patient started. The patient then uses more and more drug with less and less effect. The chronic topical use of appreciable doses of these medications can lead to the loss of cilia of the epithelial cells. Thickening of the mucosa has been noted after just five days of use [18]. Withdrawal of the topical sympathomimetic therapy is required but is often difficult to accomplish. Three methods have been advocated [17]: the simplest is to stop use in one nostril for one to two weeks, followed by stopping use in the other. Another is the use of systemic antihistamine and vasoactive amine which does not seem to produce this problem. Lastly, is the replacement by steroid treatment. Baldwin *et al.* [19] in comparing these techniques, found each to be effective. However, in patients with chronic rhinitis the replacement by topical steroid would seem to be the best choice, insofar as it allows for concurrent treatment of their underlying problem.

Some caution is required with topical nasal vasoconstrictor medications to avoid systemic symptoms, for instance in conditions where there is a risk of aggravating systemic disease including narrow angle glaucoma, hypertension and heart disease. They should not be used in people on monoamine oxidase inhibitors or tricyclic antidepressants.

A beneficial effect of fenoterol hydrobromide, a selective beta agonist, has recently been reported in allergic rhinitis [20,21]. Since it has a vasodilatory effect and initially increases nasal airway resistance, non-vascular effects were invoked to explain the results.

In summary, there is a limited but reasonably well defined short term role for vasoactive amines in the current topical treatment of rhinitis. However, the potential applications of these drugs have not yet been fully explored and there may be a broadening of their use in the future.

ANTIHISTAMINES

Bovet and Staub in 1937 discovered the first in a series of substances which protected animals from a lethal dose of histamine [22]. With the numerous systemically administered antihistamines that have been developed, topical use has received relatively little attention. The possibility that topical use might lead to sensitisation may have been a deterrent [23]. Ingested antihistamines have the benefit of simplicity of administration and the capacity to reduce symptoms in different locations, such as nose and eyes. Intranasal therapy with H_1 antagonists has received much less attention but could have the advantages of local topical therapy.

Histamine blocking agents occupy histamine receptors on cell membranes thereby blocking the effects of histamine. The antihistamines initially discovered are now designated H_1 receptors; they block mainly vasodilatation, hypersecretion, broncho-constriction, and contraction of the gut. H_2 antagonists block mainly the stimulation of gastric secretion but also tend to inhibit cardiovascular effects of histamine.

Systemic H_1 blockade has been shown to be effective in allergic rhinitis while little effect has been seen in non-allergic rhinitis [24,25]. Topical antihistamine is commonly included with alpha adrenergic agonists in nasal topical preparations. However, the effectiveness of topical H_1 blockers has only recently been tested in clinical trials. Chlorpheniramine [23] and two newer agents, azatadine [26] and levocabastine [27,28], have been shown to be effective in nasal challenges and clinical studies. Levocabastine was shown in one study to be comparable to sodium cromoglycate in low dosage in challenge testing [28]. Also, the combination of topical H_1 and H_2 blockers, chlorpheniramine and ranitidine, have shown some additive effect in relief of histamine induced nasal congestion but not sneezing or hypersecretion [29]. Some irritability and bitterness has been reported with these drugs but only with high doses and ranitidine were the effects significant. These studies are at a preliminary stage. Further drug studies with each drug alone and in combination with other modes of therapy are needed to establish the place of topical antihistamine therapy in chronic rhinitis.

ANTICHOLINERGICS

Atropine, a potent anticholinergic obtained from belladonna plants, has been used by man since ancient times. Unfortunately, it was generally used as a poison. The benefits of topical therapy were first discovered by sufferers of chronic obstructive pulmonary disease who, in keeping with their habits, found improvement when the smoke from the leaves was inhaled [30]. Parasympathetic

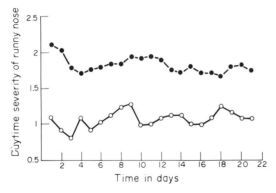

Figure 1: Daytime severity of nasal discharge during ipratropium bromide *(open circles)* and placebo treatment *(closed dots)*. Daily mean values from the diary cards of the 25 subjects are presented. There was a highly significant reduction ($p < 0.00005$) in the nasal discharge during active treatment. (From *J Allergy Clin Immunol* 1988; **80**: 274. Reprinted by kind permission of the publishers.)

(cholinergic) stimulation increases the activity of guanylate cyclase, a cell membrane associated enzyme. This catalyses the increased formation of cGMP. There is an increased release of intracellular calcium which increases the contraction of smooth muscle and facilitates glandular secretion and the release of mediators from mast cells leading to detrimental affects in the airways. Cholinergic blockers would inhibit these actions which potentially could explain an effectiveness in both upper and lower airway allergic and non-allergic disease [30,31] . Topical atropine is sufficiently absorbed to elicit multiple systemic side effects. Ipratropium bromide, a quaternary derivative of isoproyl noratropine with low lipid solubility and a low level of systemic effects, has led to renewed interest in topical anticholinergic therapy.

Numerous recent reports attest to an effectiveness in the control of profuse rhinorrhoea of vasomotor rhinitis [32–39]. The effect in rhinitis with marked hypersecretion is shown in Fig. 1 [34]. A local drying effect leading to burning, cracking, and bleeding has been reported, especially with higher doses [40]. The use of 80 μg three times a day initially, and then in decreasing frequency to find the minimum dose needed to control symptoms, appears to alleviate these problems. Systemic side effects do not seem to be an issue. Single doses of 400 μg, 5–10 times the usual dose, seem to be tolerated with only minimal systemic effects [41].

In allergic rhinitis ipratropium bromide aerosol had a suppressive effect on methacholine nasal challenge-induced hypersecretion and sneezing but no change in nasal resistance [42]. This is consistent with the expectation that any effect on smooth muscle would be a relaxation which, if anything, would be detrimental to nasal obstruction. In patients with marked hypersecretion as one of the main symptoms of allergic rhinitis, topical ipratropium bromide would seem to be worth a try as an adjunctive therapy, although clinical trials would be needed to confirm its usefulness.

Thus, there is an established role for ipratropium bromide for the syndrome of profuse watery hypersecretion of non-allergic rhinitis and possibly for allergic rhinitis. Care is required to establish the minimum dose needed to control the hypersecretion in order to avoid local side effects.

SODIUM CROMOGLYCATE

Sodium cromoglycate was developed by modification of the substance khellin, a chromone of plant origin [43]. The drug was found to prevent allergic bronchoconstriction by an apparently novel mechanism. It is known to inhibit the secretion of mast cell mediators and products of other inflammatory cells, although part of the effectiveness in asthma is probably through inhibition of reflex bronchoconstriction [44].

Sodium cromoglycate is better than placebo in treatment of allergic rhinitis [45–48]. Handelman et al. [45] in a multicentre double-blind crossover study with 104 patients showed significant benefit of the drug over a six week period with minimal side effects. Their results are summarised in Fig. 2. Minimal local irritation has been reported which often dissipates with time. Also, sodium cromoglycate has been shown to be beneficial to patients with non-allergic rhinitis with oesinophilia (NARES) syndrome [49]. It appears to have no effect in non-allergic rhinitis. In a double-blind six week trial during the ragweed season cromoglycate (2%) was shown to be superior to ingested terfenadine, a non-sedating H_1 blocker, at a dose of 120 mg/day [50]. In addition, over a four year period there was no difference in effectiveness between topical nasal sodium cromoglycate and allergen injection therapy [51]. However, seven published studies have compared topical nasal cromoglycate with topical nasal steroid; the latter was superior in six [52–57] and the two medications were equivalent in one [58] in which only 20 subjects were tested. Welsh et al. recently compared

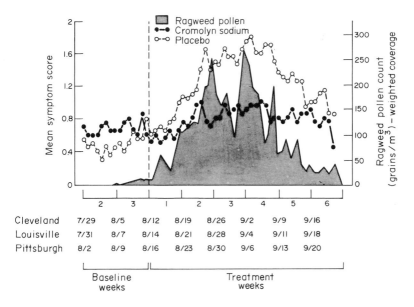

Figure 2: Daily symptoms and pollen pattern for rhinorrhoea (daytime scores). (From J *Allergy Clin Immunol*, 1977; **59**: 237–42. Reprinted by kind permission of the publishers.)

beclomethasone and flunisolide (two different topical steroids) with high dose (4%) cromoglycate; the steroids were more effective [57]. Their findings are summarised in Fig. 3. Local burning was experienced in the flunisolide group. A new flunisolide formulation which contains only 5% propylene glycol vs 20% has been found to be better tolerated [59].

In conclusion, topical cromoglycate is effective and safe in allergic rhinitis. Steroid has greater effectiveness but occasionally produces local side effects. Thus, intranasal steroid appears usually to be more advantageous as the drug of choice for allergic rhinitis. The role of cromoglycate in combination with steroid for patient failures has not been investigated clinically although some have suggested benefit from the combination [60].

Nedocromil sodium is more potent than sodium cromoglycate in inhibition of mucosal mast cell mediator release *in vitro* and is a better inhibitor of axonal reflexes. Nedocromil was shown to be superior to placebo in allergic rhinitis in two recent studies [62,63]. The place of nedocromil sodium in the topical therapy of allergic rhinitis is not yet determined.

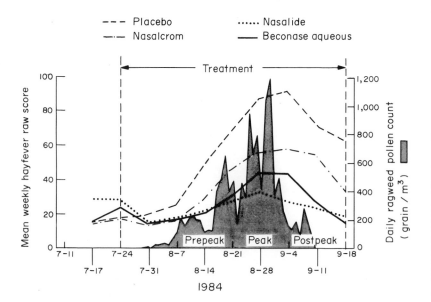

Figure 3: Mean weekly raw scores for symptoms of hay fever among 120 patients in four study groups, based on treatment: placebo, cromolyn sodium (Nasalcrom), flunisolide (Nasalide), and beclomethasone nasal solution (Beconase AQ.) Study was conducted during ragweed season in 1984. Daily ragweed pollen count is shown in shaded area. All active treatments were more effective than placebo, and the two glucocorticoids were more effective than cromolyn in preventing symptoms of hay fever. (From *Mayo Clin Proc* 1987; **62**: 130. Reprinted by kind permission of the publishers.)

In summary, sodium cromoglycate is a safe and effective therapy for allergic rhinitis but less effective than intranasal steroid. Its use in combination with other medications has not been well studied. Other cromoglycate-like drugs hold promise for the future.

NEWER EXPERIMENTAL THERAPY

With increased understanding of the pathogenesis of rhinitis, new therapies are being developed. Intracellular calcium appears to have an important role in mast cell stability. The use of a calcium channel antagonist could, therefore, be of benefit. Secher *et al.* studied the effect of topical intranasal verapamil in nasal challenges but were unable to show any benefit [64].

IgE pentapeptide (HEPP) is said to inhibit the IgE-dependent allergic reaction. Prenner has applied the peptide intranasally in a clinical trial during spring with a beneficial effect in a small number of patients [65]. Further investigation appears to be warranted.

A dipeptide N-acetyl-aspartyl-glutamic acid (NAAGA) has been shown to inhibit mast cell degranulation as well as the cytolytic effects of activated complement [66]. In initial studies there is evidence that it is effective topically in nasal allergen challenge and in treatment of seasonal allergic rhinitis [67,68]. In one study NAAGA 6% was compared to sodium cromoglycate 2%; NAAGA was found equally or more effective and just as safe [69].

SUMMARY

Rhinitis is a common cause of symptoms but is not a life-threatening disease. Therapy must be entirely free of serious adverse effects to be acceptable for long-term use. Moreover, if it is not simple to use, ongoing compliance is unlikely. Avoidance of offending substances is the best treatment of allergic rhinitis but generally this is impossible to accomplish entirely. Topical therapy generally has the inherent advantages of efficacy and particularly of systemic safety. Modern effective delivery devices and careful instruction of the patient are likely to improve results. In most cases of rhinitis, intranasal steroid alone or perhaps with preparatory saline or vasoactive amines may be the only therapy needed. There is often a place for ingested H_1 antihistamine. In patients with non-allergic rhinitis with profuse watery rhinorrhoea, topical nasal ipratropium bromide is often likely to be highly effective.

The use of combination therapy with various agents has received little formal investigation but may provide an answer in difficult cases. Despite the various treatment modalities available, there is still a place for effective new forms of therapy.

REFERENCES

1. Wright J. *A history of laryngology and rhinology*. New York: Lea and Febiger, 1914: 27–76.
2. Mygind N. Rhinitis. In: *Essential allergy*. Oxford: Blackwell Scientific Publications, 1986: 277–348.
3. Wilson R, Sykes DA, Chan KL, Cole PJ, MacKay IS. Effect of head position on the efficacy of topical treatment of chronic mucopurulent rhinosinusitis. *Thorax* 1987; **42**: 631–2.
4. Mygind N. *Nasal allergy*. Oxford: Blackwell Scientific Publications, 1979: Conventional medical treatment, 257–70.

5. Spector SL, Toshener D, Gay I, Rosenman E. Beneficial effects of propylene and polyethylene glycol and saline in the treatment of perennial rhinitis. *Clin Allergy* 1982; **12**: 187–96.
6. Bollag U, Albrecht, E, Wingert W. Medicated versus saline nose drops in the management of upper respiratory infection. *Helv paediat Acta* 1984; **39**: 341–5.
7. Meltzer EO, Schatz M, Zeiger RS. Allergic and nonallergic rhinitis. In: Middleton E, Reed CE, Ellis EF, *et al.* eds. *Allergy: principles and practice.* St Louis: CV Mosby, 1988: 1253–89.
8. Ophir D, Elad Y, Dolev Z, Geller-Bernstein C. Effects of inhaled humidified warm air on nasal patency and nasal symptoms in allergic rhinitis. *Ann Allergy* 1988; **60**: 239–42.
9. Yerushalmi A, Karman S, Lwoff A. Treatment of perennial allergic rhinitis by local hyperthermia. *Proc Natl Acad Sci USA* 1982; **79**: 4766–9.
10. Meffler C, Meffler F. *A history of medicine.* New York: The Blakiston Co. 1947: 178.
11. Kully BM. The use and abuse of nasal vasoconstrictor medications. *JAMA* 1945; **127**: 307.
12. Stride RD. Nasal decongestant therapy. *Br J Clin Pract* 1967; **21**: 541–8.
13. Barger G, Dall HH. Chemical structure and sympathomimetic action of amines. *J Physiol (Lond)* 1910; **41**: 19.
14. Petrusson B. Treatment with xylometazoline (Otrivin) nosedrops over a six-week period. *Rhinology* 1981; **19**(3): 167–72.
15. Simons FER. Allergic rhinitis: recent advances. *Ped Clin N Am* 1988; **35**: 1053–74.
16. Toohill RJ, Lehman RH, Grossman TW, Belson TP. Rhinitis medicamentosa. *Larynogoscope* 1981; **91**: 1614–20.
17. Black MJ, Remsen KA. Rhinitis medicamentosa. *Can Med Assoc J* 1980; **122**: 881–4.
18. Ryan RE. Vasomotor rhinitis medicamentosa viewed histologically. *Proc Staff Meet Mayo Clin* 1947; **22**: 113.
19. Baldwin RL. Rhinitis medicamentosa: (An approach to treatment). *J Med Assoc State Ala* 1977; **47**: 33.
20. Ford RM. Fenoterol hydrobromide (Berotec, Th 1165a) 0.1% solution in the treatment of allergic rhinitis. *Ann Allergy* 1980; **44**: 112–5.
21. Schumacher MJ. Effect of a β-adrenergic agonist, fenoterol, on nasal sensitivity to allergen. *J Allergy Clin Immunol* 1980; **66**: 33–6.
22. Goodman LS, Gilman A. *The pharmacological basis of therapeutics.* New York: Macmillan, 1985: 618.
23. Kirkegaard J, Secher C, Borum P, Mygind N. Inhibition of histamine-induced nasal symptoms by the H_1 antihistamine chlorpheniramine maleate: demonstration of topical effect. *Br J Dis Chest* 1983; **77**: 113–22.
24. Lieberman P. Rhinitis: allergic and nonallergic. *Hosp Pract* 1988; June: 117–45.
25. Simons FER, Simons KJ. H_1 receptor antagonist treatment of chronic rhinitis. *J Allergy Clin Immunol* 1988; **81**: 975– 80.
26. Togias A, Proud D, Kagey-Sobotka A, Norman P, Lichtenstein L, Naclerio R. The effect of a topical tricyclic antihistamine on the response of the nasal mucosa to challenge with cold, dry air and histamine. *J Allergy Clin Immunol* 1987; **79**: 599–604.
27. Bende M, Pipkorn U. Topical levocabastine, a selective H_1 antagonist, in seasonal allergic rhinoconjunctivitis. *Allergy* 1987; **42**: 512–5.
28. Kolly M, Pecoud A. Comparison of levocabastine, a new selective H_1-receptor antagonist, and disodium cromoglycate, in a nasal provocation test with allergen. *Br J Clin Pharm* 1986; **22**: 389–94.
29. Secher C, Kirkegaard J, Borum P, Maansson A, Osterhammel P, Mygind N. Significance of H_1 and H_2 receptors in the human nose: rationale for topical use of combined antihistamine preparations. *J Allergy Clin Immunol* 1982; **70**: 211–8.
30. Massey KL, Gotz VP. Ipratropium bromide. *Drug Intell Clin Pharmacy* 1985; **19**: 5–12.

31. Mygind N. *Nasal allergy*. Oxford: Blackwell Scientific Publications, 1979; Topical ipratropium—a new approach in rhinitis treatment, 333–42.
32. Sjogren I, Juhasz J. Ipratropium in the treatment of patients with perennial rhinitis. *Allergy* 1984; **39**: 457–61.
33. Knight A, Kazim F, Salvatori VA. A trial of intranasal Atrovent versus placebo in the treatment of vasomotor rhinitis. *Ann Allergy* 1986; **57**: 348–54.
34. Dolovich J, Kennedy L, Vickerson F, Kazim F. Control of the hypersecretion of vasomotor rhinitis by topical ipratropium bromide. *J Allergy Clin Immunol* 1987; **80**: 274–8.
35. Borum P. Nasal disorders and anticholinergic therapy. *Postgraduate Med J* 1987; **63**(1): 61–8.
36. Malmberg H, Grahne B, Holopainen E, Binder E. Ipratropium (Atrovent) in the treatment of vasomotor rhinitis of elderly patients. *Clin Otolaryngol* 1983; **8**: 273–6.
37. Bok HE, Van Wijingaarden HA, Cornelissen PJG. Intranasal ipratropium bromide for paroxysmal rhinorrhoea. *Eur J Respir Dis* 1983; **64**(128): 486–9.
38. Borum P, Mygind N, Larsen FS. Intranasal ipratropium: a new treatment for perennial rhinitis. *Clin Otolaryngol* 1979; **4**: 407– 11.
39. Borum P, Olsen L, Winther B, Mygind N. Ipratropium nasal spray: A new treatment for rhinorrhea in the common cold. *Am Rev Respir Dis* 1981; **123**: 418–20.
40. Kirkegaard J, Mygind N, Molgaard F, *et al.* Ordinary and high-dose ipratropium in perennial nonallergic rhinitis. *J Allergy Clin Immunol* 1987; **79**: 585–90.
41. Groth S, Dirksen H, Mygind N. The absence of systemic side-effects from high doses of ipratropium in the nose. *Eur J Respir Dis* 1983; **64**(128): 490–3.
42. Sanwikarja S, Schmitz PIM, Dieges PH. The effect of locally applied ipratropium aerosol on the nasal methacholine challenge in patients with allergic and non-allergic rhinitis. *Ann Allergy* 1986; **56**: 162–7.
43. Goodman LS, Gilman A. *The pharmacological basis of therapeutics* . New York: Macmillan, 1985: 616.
44. Church MK, Warner JO. Sodium cromoglycate and related drugs. *Clin Allergy* 1985; **15**: 311–20.
45. Handelman NI, Friday GA, Schwartz HJ, *et al.* Cromolyn sodium nasal solution in the prophylactic treatment of pollen-induced seasonal allergic rhinitis. A tri-city study of efficacy and safety. *J Allergy Clin Immunol* 1977; **59**: 237–42.
46. Leiferman KM, Yunginger JW, Larson JB, Gleich GJ. The effect of cromolyn sodium powder as a treatment for ragweed pollinosis. *J Allergy Clin Immunol* 1975; **56**(6): 482–90.
47. Chandra RK, Heresi G, Woodford G. Double-blind controlled crossover trial of 4% intranasal sodium cromoglycate solution in patients with seasonal allergic rhinitis. *Ann Allergy* 1982; **49**: 131– 4.
48. Van Niekerk CH. Sodium cromoglycate/chlorpheniramine and sodium cromoglycate nasal sprays in the treatment of seasonal rhinitis. *S Afr Med J* 1985; **67**: 801–3.
49. Nelson BL, Jacobs RL. Response of the nonallergic rhinitis with eosinophilia (NARES) syndrome to 4% cromolyn sodium nasal solution. *J Allergy Clin Immunol* 1982; **70**: 125–8.
50. Lindsay-Miller ACM, Chambers A. Group comparative trial of cromolyn sodium and terfenadine in the treatment of seasonal allergic rhinitis. *Ann Allergy* 1987; **58**: 28–32.
51. Andersen NH, Jeppesen F, Schioler T, Osterballe O. Treatment of hay fever with sodium cromoglycate, hyposensitization, or a combination. *Allergy* 1987; **42**: 343–51.
52. Frankland AW, Walker SR. A comparison of intranasal betamethasone valerate and sodium cromoglycate in seasonal allergic rhinitis. *Clin Allergy* 1975; **5**: 295–300.
53. Hillas J, Booth RJ, Somerfield S, Morton R, Avery J, Wilson JD. A comparative

trial of intra-nasal beclomethasone dipropionate and sodium cromoglycate in patients with chronic perennial rhinitis. *Clin Allergy* 1980; **10**: 253–8.

54. Tandon MK, Strahan EG. Double-blind crossover trial comparing beclomethasone dipropionate and sodium cromoglycate in perennial allergic rhinitis. *Clin Allergy* 1980; **10**: 459–62.

55. Brown HM, Engler C, English JR. A comparative trial of flunisolide and sodium cromoglycate nasal sprays in the treatment of seasonal allergic rhinitis. *Clin Allergy* 1981; **11**: 169–73.

56. Bjerrum P, Illum P. Treatment of seasonal allergic rhinitis with budesonide and disodium cromoglycate. *Allergy* 1985; **40**: 65–9.

57. Welsh PW, Stricker WE, Chu C-P, *et al*. Efficacy of beclomethasone nasal solution, flunisolide, and cromolyn in relieving symptoms of ragweed allergy. *Mayo Clin Proc* 1987; **62**: 125–34.

58. Chatterjee SS, Nassar WY, Wilson O, Butler AG. Intra-nasal beclomethasone dipropionate and intra-nasal sodium cromoglycate: a comparative trial. *Clin Allergy* 1974; **4**: 343–8.

59. Greenbaum J, Leznoff A, Schulz J, Mazza J, Tobe A, Miller D. Comparative tolerability of two formulations of Rhinalar (flunisolide) nasal spray in patients with seasonal allergic rhinitis. *Ann Allergy* 1988; **61**: 305–10.

60. Pelikan Z. The effects of disodium cromoglycate (DSCG) and beclomethasone dipropionate (BDA) on the delayed nasal mucosa response to allergen challenge. *Ann Allergy* 1984; **52**: 111–24.

61. Gonzalez JP, Brogden RN. Nedocromil sodium. A preliminary review of its pharmacodynamic and pharmocokinetic properties, and therapeutic efficacy in the treatment of reversible obstructive airways disease. *Drugs* 1987; **34**: 560–77.

62. Corrado OJ, Gomez E, Baldwin DL, Clague JE, Davies RJ. The effect of nedocromil sodium on nasal provocation with allergen. *J Allergy Clin Immunol* 1987; **80**: 218–22.

63. Ruhno J, Denburg J, Dolovich J. Intranasal nedocromil sodium in the treatment of ragweed-allergic rhinitis. *J Allergy Clin Immunol* 1988; **81**: 570–4.

64. Secher C, Brofeldt S, Mygind N. Intranasal verapamil in allergen-induced rhinitis. *Allergy* 1983; **38**: 565–70.

65. Prenner BM. Double-blind placebo-controlled trial of intranasal IgE pentapeptide. *Ann Allergy* 1987; **58**: 332–35.

66. Etievant B, Leluc B, David B. *In vitro* inhibition of the classical and alternate pathways of activation of human complement by N acetyl aspartyl glutamic acid (NAAGA). *Agents Actions* 1988; **24**: 137–44.

67. Ghaem A. A preliminary evaluation of the effect of N-acetyl-aspartyl-glutamate on pollen nasal challenge as measured by rhinomanometry and symptomatology. *Allergy* 1987; **42**: 626–30.

68. Paupe J, Paupe G, Brunet-Langot D, Dalayeun H. Activité d'un nouvel anti-allergique, l'acide N-acetyl aspartyl glutamique, dans les rhinites allergiques de l'enfant. *Extrait de Revue Francaise d'allergologie* 1988; **3**: 241–5.

69. Blamoutier J, Luyckx J. A double-blind cross-over study comparing N-acetyl-aspartyl glutamic acid (NAAGA) with disodium cromoglycate (DSCG) in the treatment of perennial allergic rhinitis. *Acta Therapeutica* 1988; **14**: 145–57.

Chapter 11

TOPICAL MEDICAL MANAGEMENT OF ALLERGIC CONDITIONS OF THE NOSE
Part 2: INTRANASAL STEROIDS

Ian S. Mackay

INTRODUCTION

The cardinal symptoms of rhinitis are sneezing, watery rhinorrhoea and nasal obstruction resulting from the inflammation of the respiratory mucous membranes. A cure for these symptoms remains the ultimate goal for both patients and practitioners. However, as yet the best we can hope to achieve for the majority of patients is to control the symptoms without producing side-effects.

The most effective antiinflammatory drugs available are the corticosteroids. Given systemically in large doses they will usually abolish all the symptoms but with an unacceptable risk of side-effects. That is not to say, however, that they do not have any place in the treatment of allergic rhinitis. Indeed they may well have an important role in controlling severe seasonal symptoms of short duration, or to gain control prior to prescribing topical treatment.

Topical steroids should offer the maximum local effect with the minimum of side-effects and indeed the topical use of hydrocortisone snuff [1] and prednisolone snuff [2] used in the 1950s appeared to be of little or no advantage compared to the systemic route, as both resulted in depression of the hypothalamic-pituitary-adrenal (HPA) axis. Dexamethasone was introduced in the 1960s and shown to be effective in the treatment of both seasonal and perennial allergic rhinitis [3]. In large doses this too will affect the HPA axis as it is absorbed and is not inactivated in the liver. In the 1970s, however, beclomethasone dipropionate (BDP) was introduced, which was shown to have no or minimal systemic effect while maintaining its effect locally [4].

INDICATIONS

Seasonal allergy

The best example of seasonal allergy in the United Kingdom is hayfever. Other allergies, however, may be seasonal in that a seasonal increase in symptoms may be experienced by patients suffering from allergies to moulds or mites in certain climates.

This group of patients respond particularly well to topical corticosteroids and trials have shown complete control of all nasal symptoms in up to 90% of patients [5].

Perennial allergic rhinitis

Perennial allergic rhinitis is more difficult to control than seasonal allergic rhinitis. It is important that these patients should be controlled with topically acting corticosteroids with minimal systemic activity as these patients will require long-term maintenance treatment and are the very patients in whom it is best to avoid systemic medication which could influence the HPA-axis. Fortunately, although this group is less easily controlled than the systemic group, many trials have shown satisfactory results particularly in the atopic [skin test positive] group [6].

Non-allergic (vasomotor) rhinitis

Patients with perennial symptoms of rhinitis, with nasal blockage, sneezing and watery rhinorrhoea throughout the year who are found to have negative skin tests, negative challenges, and no history of allergy are sometimes grouped together under the heading of vasomotor rhinitis. This group probably represents a variety of different aetiologies:- emotional, hyper-active, hormonal, cystic fibrosis, ciliary dyskinesia, etc. Fortunately some of these patients will still respond to topical corticosteroids. If a nasal smear is taken and eosinophils are seen, it is thought that the patient may be more likely to respond to corticosteroids though the presence of eosinophils may vary from time to time, even in the same patient [7]. Even in the absence of eosinophilia, a trial with steroids would be worthwhile, providing that this does not replace a thorough investigation to attempt to find the underlying cause.

Infective rhinosinusitis

Inflammation of the nose and paranasal sinuses leads to swelling of the respiratory ciliated mucosa which quickly blocks the natural ostia. This may be followed by secondary infection which results in further inflammation and stasis. Treatment should be aimed at interrupting the vicious circle which would otherwise result in progressive tissue damage. Treatment should be aimed at: (1) The microbial flora—using antimicrobial agents. (2) The tissue damaging inflammatory response—using topical antiinflammatory agents; and (3) Improving clearance—with topical washings and possibly surgery to improve drainage and ventilation [8].

Nasal polyps

The aetiology and pathogenesis of nasal polyps is poorly understood and indeed there are probably several entirely different mechanisms responsible. For example, the pathogenesis involved in nasal polyps occurring in cystic fibrosis, aspirin induced asthmatics and atopic asthmatics may well be entirely different. However, up to 60% of nasal polyps will respond to topical corticosteroids providing these are applied in a position designed to increase exposure of the mucosal lining of the ethmoidal sinuses [see below] [9]. In the study undertaken at The Brompton Hospital we were unable to identify any discriminant for response or non-response to betamethasone.

Granulomatous conditions

Granular mucosa is seen in various conditions in the nose such as sarcoid, or Wegener's granulomatosis, and patients with AIDS may develop a similar appearance with granulation tissue, blood clots and crusts. With all these conditions it is vital to make a definitive diagnosis undertaking chest X-rays, blood tests and mucosal biopsies. The treatment will be of the underlying cause whenever possible, but the granulomatous mucosa will often respond to topical corticosteroids and when treating sarcoid, if this is limited to the nasal mucosa, it may be possible to reduce significantly the systemic dosage of steroids [10].

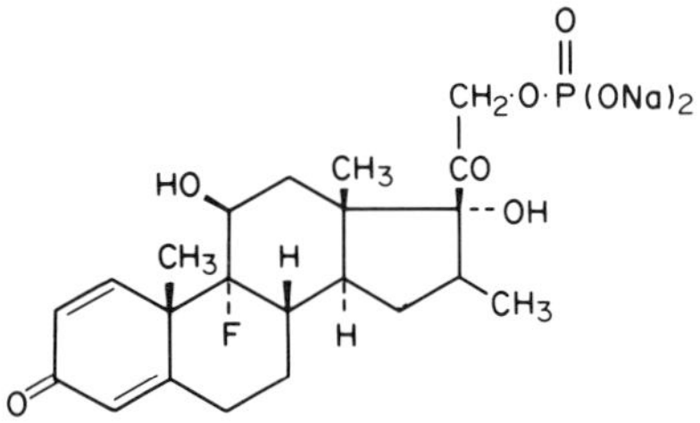

Betamethasone Sodium Phosphate

Figure 1

DRUGS AVAILABLE

Betamethasone

Betamethasone (Fig. 1) is administered in drop form and, providing this is used in an advantageous position, penetrance can be excellent. It is particularly effective in the treatment of nasal polyps, and can be useful in controlling mucopurulent rhinorrhoea in patients with chronic infective symptoms.

It is absorbed and can be expected to have a systemic effect: indeed it may be because of this that it is so effective in gaining control of symptoms in the initial phase. The total dose of steroid however is relatively low. If two drops are taken each side twice daily, i.e. eight drops a day, this is equivalent to 1.15 mg of prednisolone daily (10 ml of Betnesol contains 10 mg of betamethasone sodium phosphate. One drop of Betnesol from a nasal drop bottle is approximately 0.028 ml [11], and 0.75 mg of betamethasone is equivalent to 5 mg of prednisolone [12]). It is not thought that this dose is likely to cause significant side-effects; nonetheless it is better to avoid long-term usage of betamethasone and to replace this with beclomethasone dipropionate to maintain any improvement.

Dexamethasone

Dexamethasone phosphate (Fig. 2) was one of the first topical steroids available as an aerosol. It is still available in many countries including the United Kingdom and the United States. In the United Kingdom, it is marketed as an aerosol spray containing dexamethasone, neomycin and tramazoline hydrochloride, the

186

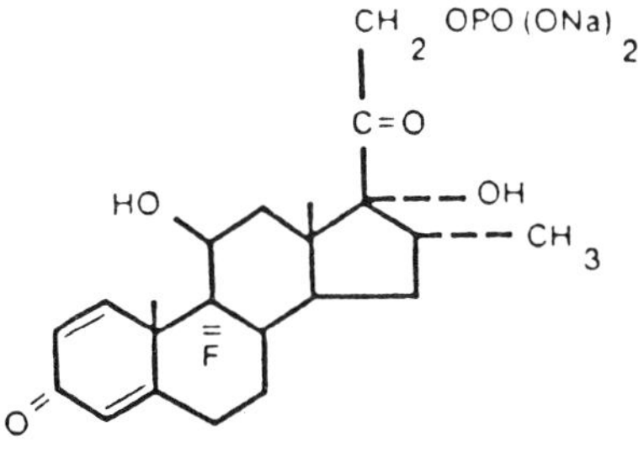

Dexamethasone Sodium Phosphate

Figure 2

latter being a decongestant. The topical use of antibiotics in the nose is of doubtful value, even when treating chronic mucopurulent rhinosinusitis [13]. Topical decongestants are not recommended for long-term use and since dexamethasone is absorbed and does have a systemic effect, the long-term use of this spray is not recommended. Nevertheless, it does appear to have a useful role in controlling symptoms of chronic rhinosinusitis and, out of the 40 patients receiving active treatment in the Brompton trial [13] 26 (65%) patients found that application of this four times daily for two weeks was beneficial compared with two patients out of 10 (20%) in the placebo group.

Beclomethasone dipropionate

Initial trials on asthmatic patients using beclomethasone dipropionate (BDP) (Fig. 3) revealed that a daily dose of 400 μg had an anti-asthmatic effect approximating that of 5–10 mg of prednisolone taken orally without affecting plasma cortisol [14].

BDP was introduced for topical use in the nose in 1973 [5]; initially introduced as a freon propelled metered-dose aerosol, this was the first topical steroid which clearly demonstrated effective topical activity without systemic effects.

Flunisolide

Flunisolide (Fig. 4) was introduced in 1976 [15]. This is delivered by a mechanical pump with the active ingredient dissolved in

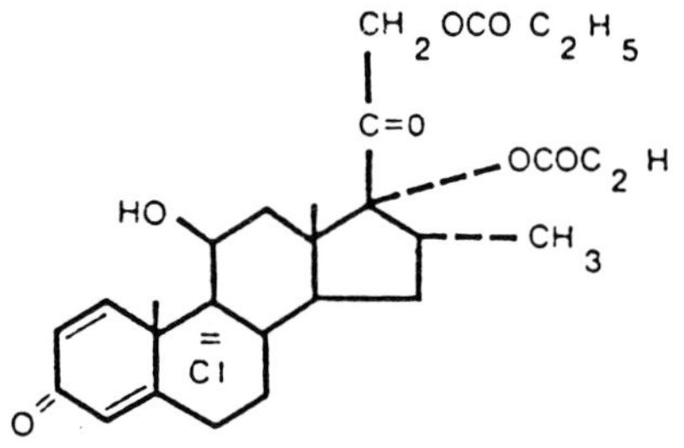

Beclomethasone Dipropionate

Figure 3

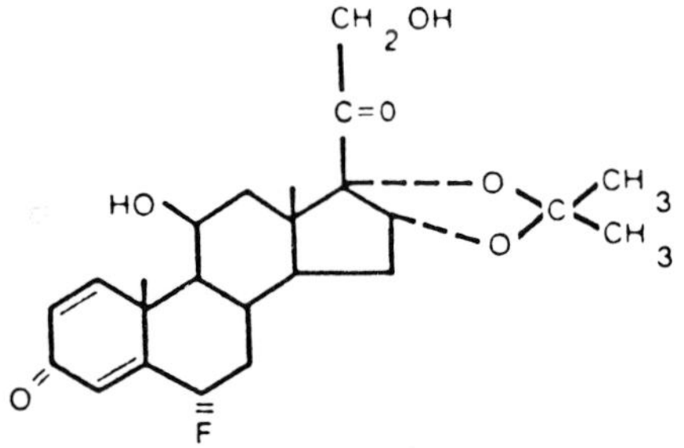

Flunisolide

Figure 4

polyethylene glycol, propylene glycol and water. Similar in potency to BDP, it too is effective when used topically and has no adverse effect on the HPA-axis.

Budesonide

Budesonide (Fig. 5) was introduced in 1980 [16]: similar in action to the two topical steroids described above, it is said to be slightly more potent topically when judged by the cutaneous vasoconstriction test for anti-inflammatory activity [17].

Fluticasone

The latest of the topical steroids to be used is fluticasone propionate (Fig. 6) which will be available as an aqueous nasal spray for

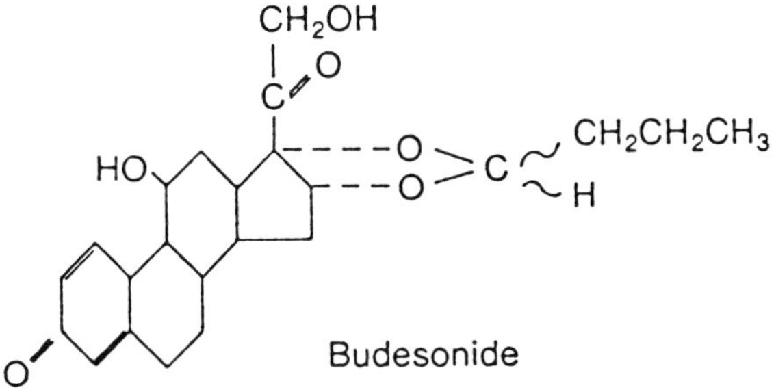

Budesonide

Figure 5

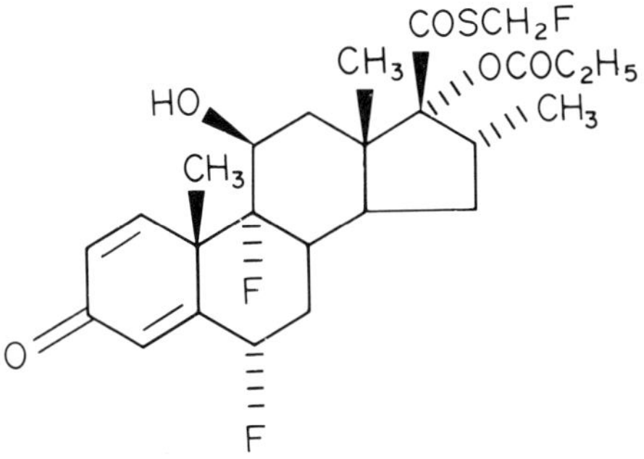

Figure 6

administration to the nasal mucosa using a metering atomising pump. At the time of writing this chapter, clinical trials with this preparation have not yet been completed. Early results however are very promising.

APPLICATION

Dosage

The daily dosage of beclomethasone dipropionate used in controlling asthma was initially 400 µg [4] and, somewhat empirically, this dosage was advocated for topical use in the nose. The Brompton Hospital/Medical Research Council Collaborative Trial [6] found 400 µg more effective than 200 µg in controlling the symptoms of allergic rhinitis though increasing the dosage above this level to 800 μg was shown by Malm and Wihl to be no more effective [18]. Siegel *et al.* also confirmed that there was little to be gained from increasing the dosage above 400 μg [19].

In practice, however, the dose often needs to be varied upwards or downwards in the individual patient to maintain control, and dosages as low as 50 μg per day may well control patients with perennial symptoms while hayfever sufferers may need to use as much as 1200 μg daily on days when the pollen counts are particularly high [20].

Frequency

One of the major advantages of topical steroids over sodium cromoglycate (SCG) is that symptoms can usually be controlled with twice daily application [21], whereas SCG may need to be used four or five times daily in order to be effective. Compliance with the topical steroids is therefore likely to be better.

Betamethasone drops are also used on a twice-daily regime though this can usually be reduced to a once-daily dose once the symptoms have been controlled.

Dexamethasone, if combined with a decongestant, may be used in a reducing dosage starting with a dose of two puffs to each nostril four times a day and reducing to two puffs to each nostril once or twice daily over a period of two weeks. It is better to avoid long-term usage and to change to BDP or an equivalent topical corticosteroid for maintenance.

Propellant

BDP and budesonide are available as either a freon-propelled spray or in an aqueous solution in a mechanically operated pump. Flunisolide is available in a similar mechanically operated pump but dissolved in a mixture of polyethylene glycols, propylene glycol and water.

Freon (apart from the fact that it may be dissolving the earth's ozone layer) has the possible disadvantage that it may cause dryness of the mucous membranes. Some patients complain that polyethylene and propylene glycol cause stinging, particularly in the initial stages of treatment but this disadvantage may be outweighed by the beneficial effect which the glycols themselves have in the treatment of perennial rhinitis [22].

Clinical trials have failed to show any significant difference in efficacy between the various vehicles [23, 24] and, at the end of the day, patient preference is the more important factor. The freon-propelled sprays are convenient and simple to use; if this results in dryness then it is worth a trial with the polyethylene propylene glycols. If this causes unacceptable stinging, the aqueous solutions in mechanically operated pumps may be more acceptable.

Dexamethasone (combined with antibiotic and decongestant) is delivered via an aerosol spray. Betamethasone drops are made up in 5 ml and 10 ml plastic squeezable bottles designed to be inverted and squeezed gently to deliver one drop at a time. It may be difficult for some patients to be certain how many drops they used unless these are administered by someone else. If this is not possible, it may aid the patient to keep the bottle in a fridge or cool place so that they can feel the drops as they enter the nose.

Penetrance

Mygind has shown that the freon-propelled sprays reach only a limited area of the nasal mucosa [25] and it was with this in mind that the mechanical pumps were introduced which were shown to result in a better distribution within the nasal cavity. These experiments, however, were carried out on models of the nasal cavity and almost certainly do not represent the situation in real life, as the mucociliary mechanism would result in the particles being moved backwards towards the nasopharynx, rapidly spreading the deposition posteriorly. At the same time however, this mechanism will also clear the topical corticosteroids which will disappear from the nose within 60 minutes [26].

The key area of the nose is the middle meatus. It is here that the maxillary sinuses, the ethmoidal sinuses and the frontal sinuses drain, and blockage of the ethmoids will predispose to sinus infection. It is difficult for freon-propelled or mechanically pumped sprays to reach this area, particularly if there is swelling of the mucosa of the middle and inferior turbinates or nasal polyps. It is in this situation that nasal drops instilled into the nose in the head down position are more likely to succeed. The head downwards and backwards position has been advocated by Mygind [27] (Fig. 7). Studies undertaken by the author using radio-opaque drops,

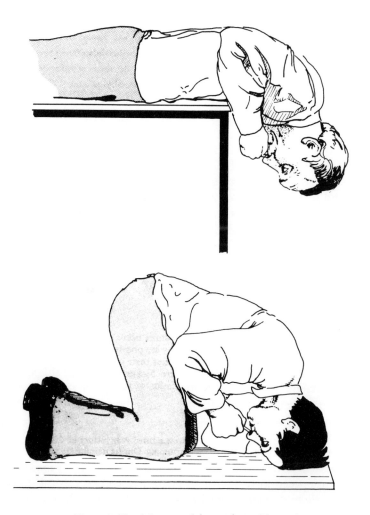

Figure 7: Head down and forwards position.

revealed the head downwards and forwards position resulted in the optimum position as far as drops penetrating the ethmoidal region and clinically, this has been shown to be very effective [28] . Unless patients are specifically instructed to use one of these two positions they are likely to instill the drops in the standing and head back position which results in the drops running down the floor of the nose into the throat where they are swallowed and since the systemic effect is negligible, little or no benefit is obtained.

COMPLICATIONS

Mygind, in his excellent book on nasal allergy, has classified the potential side-effects of topical steroids as bleeding, infection or atrophy.

Bleeding

This can be a problem in patients treated with topical steroids. Certainly, examination of the nose of patients using topical steroids will frequently reveal haemorrhagic areas in the anterior part of the nose, though very rarely is there any evidence of bleeding posteriorly. As many as 5% of patients may complain of specks of blood in the nasal secretions.

It has been suggested that this is due to excessive dryness of the nasal mucosa anteriorly rather than any specific effect of the steroids. Topical steroids used on the skin may cause fragility of the blood vessels due to steroid suppression of the fibroblasts and inhibition of collagen synthesis. In the nose, however, this seems to be less of a problem and this may be due to the fact that topical preparations are constantly being cleared by the mucociliary transport mechanism.

In some cases, it may be due to the action of the applicator rather than the medication itself and this is particularly true if there is any deviation of the nasal septum in the region of the valve, when it is prone to vestibulitis secondary to the drying effect of eddies of air currents, added to this is the effect of direct trauma from the applicator.

In cases such as this it is sometimes helpful to use topical steroid drops: either betamethasone or aqueous beclomethasone. The latter can be removed from the mechanical pump and instilled from a dropper bottle in the head prone position. It is however preferable to correct the deviation of the septum by undertaking septal surgery as this in itself may well contribute to the patient's symptoms, particularly nasal obstruction.

Although bleeding is not uncommon, it is very rarely troublesome and few patients stop treatment on account of this. Occasionally, however it may be necessary to stop the treatment for a few days and the use of a topical cream or ointment may be beneficial.

Intranasal corticosteroid injections were advocated as long ago as 1952 and excellent results have been reported. Complications, however, have been reported, the most serious of which is permanent visual loss [29]. The mechanism for this has been postulated as a vasoconstrictive or embolic phenomenon via the rich anastomoses between the ophthalmic artery and branches of the sphenopalatine artery.

Infection

Pharyngeal candidiasis is a common complication of inhaled steroids in the treatment of asthma. It is rare however to find evidence of fungal infections in the nose following even long-term treatment with topical steroids in the nose. It has been suggested that this is due to the excellent clearance mechanisms in the nose and paranasal sinuses. However, it seems likely that there are other explanations for this as the constant production of saliva and swallowing should remove inhaled steroids from the pharynx equally fast.

One might expect patients on topical nasal steroids to be more prone to upper respiratory tract infection due to bacteria and viruses, including the common cold. In practice, however, this does not appear to occur and many patients comment on the fact that they appear to suffer fewer upper respiratory tract infections while continuing treatment. This may be due to improved nasal mucociliary clearance and drainage particularly in the middle meatal ethmoidal complex.

Potentially pathogenic bacteria were found in six out of 32 cases treated with topical steroids for one year compared with five out of 30 normals in a matched control group [27]. IgA concentration in nasal secretions were unaltered in patients treated for one year [30].

Atrophy

It is accepted that long-term treatment with topical steroids may lead to atrophy of the skin but this does not occur in the bronchial or nasal mucosa.

Temporary dryness of the nasal mucosa may be observed but this will quickly resolve if the medication is stopped for a short time. Despite the fact that BPD has now been used for 15 years and in many patients, on a long-term basis, irreversible damage or permanent atrophic changes have not been reported.

In Mygind's long-term trial of patients treated with BDP for nasal polyps, pre- and post-treatment nasal biopsies were taken at one year and examined both under the light microscope and the scanning electron microscope. There was no evidence of atrophic rhinitis.

Systemic complications

Many practitioners are needlessly afraid that topical steroids may lead to systemic side-effects. There is now considerable evidence that BDP and similar topical steroids used in the recommended dose are effective locally and have no systemic side-effects.

COMPARISONS WITH OTHER TREATMENT

Sodium cromoglycate

There have been many trials which demonstrate the effectiveness of SCG [31] in controlling nasal symptoms. It has the advantage that there are no known side-effects, but needs to be used frequently (four to six times daily) in order to be effective. It should be used prophylactically. Trials comparing topical steroids with SCG show the former to be more effective in controlling the nasal symptoms, although it is useful in controlling eye symptoms [32–37].

Nedocromil sodium, has similar properties to SCG but initial studies suggest that it may be more effective in controlling nasal symptoms including that of nasal obstruction.

Antihistamines

Antihistamines have been the mainstay of treatment for allergic rhinitis for many years; until recently, however, they were associated with an unacceptable degree of sedation. This changed with the introduction of the newer H_1 antagonists (terfenadine, astemizole and cetirizine) which are very effective and non-sedating. Topical steroids have been shown to be more effective than antihistamines in controlling the symptoms of rhinitis. In particular, nasal obstruction responds better, though a combination of topical steroids and antihistamines is especially effective [38, 39].

Anticholinergics

Topical ipratropium bromide is particularly helpful in controlling watery rhinorrhoea. It is less helpful in managing the other symptoms of nasal allergy but has an important role in treating watery rhinorrhoea in perennial rhinitis not responding to topical steroids.

Vasoconstrictors

Topical and systemic vasoconstrictors may be beneficial in controlling nasal obstruction, but systemic vasoconstrictors may be associated with unwanted side-effects (headache, tachycardia, dysrhythmias, etc) and topical vasoconstrictors may cause rebound and should only be used on a short-term basis. They may, however, have a useful role in aiding penetrance of topical steroids or other medication in the initial stages of treatment.

CONCLUSION

Topical corticosteroids are extremely effective in controlling the symptoms of seasonal and perennial allergic rhinitis as well as the symptoms of non-allergic rhinitis. They play an important role in the management of nasal polyposis and have been shown to reduce the rate of recurrence of polyps following surgery. There is no evidence that, used in the recommended dosage, even for long-term maintenance of symptoms, there are any serious side-effects.

REFERENCES

1. Foulds WS, Greaves DP, Herxheimer H, Kingdom LG. Hydrocortisone in the treatment of allergic conjunctivitis, allergic rhinitis and bronchial asthma. *Lancet* 1957; i: 234–5.
2. Godfrey, MP, Maunsell K, Pearson RSE. Prednisone snuff in hayfever—a controlled trial. *Lancet* 1957; i: 767–9.
3. Boxer HM. The topical administration of corticosteroids to nasal and bronchial mucous membranes: Problems and solutions. *Proc Inst Med Chicago* 1962; **24**: 115–9.
4. Brown HM, Storey C, George WHS. Beclomethasone dipropionate: A new steroid aerosol for the treatment of allergic asthma. *Br Med J* 1972; **1**: 585–90.
5. Mygind N. Local effect of intranasal beclomethasone dipropionate aerosol in hay fever. *Br Med J* 1973; **4**: 464–6.
6. Brompton Hospital/Medical Research Council Collaborative Trial. Double-blind

trial comparing two dosage schedules of beclomethasone dipropionate in the treatment of perennial rhinitis for twelve months. *Clin Allergy* 1980; **10**: 239–51.

7. Whelan CFA. Problems in the examination of nasal smears in allergic rhinitis. *J Laryngol Otol* 1980; **94**: 399–404.

8. Mackay IS. Rhinitis and sinusitis *Br J Dis Chest* 1988; **82**: 1.

9. Chalton R, Mackay I, Wilson R, Cole P. Double-blind placebo controlled trial of betamethasone nasal drops for nasal polyposis. *Br Med J* 1985; **281**: 788.

10. Wilson R, Lund V, Sweatman M, Mackay IS, Mitchell D. Upper respiratory tract involvement in sarcoidosis and its management. *Eur Respir J* 1988; **1**: 269–72.

11. *British National Formulary* No 16, 1988; 244.

12. Glaxo Medical Information Dept.

13. Sykes DA, Wilson R, Chan KL, Mackay IS, Cole PJ. Relative importance of antibiotic and improved clearance in topical treatment of chronic mucopurulent rhinosinusitis. *Lancet* 1986; **ii**: 359.

14. Clark TJH. Effect of beclomethasone dipromionate delivered by aerosol in patients with asthma. *Lancet* 1972; **1**: 1361.

15. Turkeltaub PC, Norman PS, Crepea S. Treatment of ragweed hayfever with an intranasal spray containing flunisolide, a new synthetic corticosteroid. *J Allergy Clin Immunol* 1976; **58**: 597–606.

16. Pipkorn U, Rundcrantz H, Lindqvist N. Budesonide—a new nasal steroid . *Rhinology* 1980; **18**: 171–5.

17. Johansson S-A, Andersson K-E, Brattsand R, Gruvstad E, Hedner P. Topical and systemic glucocorticoid potencies of budesonide, beclomethasone dipropionate and prednisolone in man. *Eur J Respir Dis* 1982; **63** (Suppl 122): 74–82.

18. Malm L, Wihl J-A. Intranasal beclomethasone dipropionate in vasomotor rhinitis. *Acta Allergol* 1976; **31**: 227–38.

19. Siegel SC, Katz R, Rachelefsky GS, *et al*. Multicentric study of beclomethasone dipropionate nasal aerosol in adults with seasonal allergic rhinitis. *J Allergy Clin Immunol* 1982; **69**: 345– 53.

20. Pipkorn U, Norman PS, Middleton E Jr. In: Mygind N, Weeke B, eds. *Topical steroids in allergic and vasomotor rhinitis: clinical aspects.* Copenhagen, Munksgaard: 1985.

21. Munch E, Gomez G, Harris C, *et al*. An open comparison of dosage frequencies of beclomethasone dipropionate in seasonal allergic rhinitis. *Clin Allergy* 1981; **1**, 303–9.

22. Spector SL, Toshener D, Gay I, Roseman E. Beneficial effect of propylene and polyethylene glycol and saline in the treatment of perennial rhinitis. *Clin Allergy* 1976; **6**: 369–72.

23. Trander K, Geterud A, Lindqvist N, Pipkorn U. Comparison of two intranasal preparations of budesonide in the treatment of seasonal allergic rhinitis. *Clin Otolaryngol* 1984; **9**: 235–41.

24. Langan CE, Boyd G. Comparison of two intranasal preparations of beclomethasone dipropionate (abstract). *Folia Allergol Immunol Clin* 1983; **30** (Suppl 4): 102.

25. Mygind N, Vesterhauge S. Aerosol distribution in the nose. *Rhinology* 1978; **16**: 79–88.

26. Martin LE, Harrison C, Tanner TJN. Metabolism of beclomethasone dipropionate by animals and man. *Postgrad Med J* 1975; **51**: 11–20.

27. Mygind N. *Nasal allergy*. Oxford, England: Blackwell Scientific, 1978.

28. Wilson R, Sykes DA, Chan KL, Cole PJ, Mackay IS. Head position on efficacy of topical treatment of chronic mucopurulent rhinosinusitis. *Thorax* 1987; **42**: 631–2.

29. Mabry RL. Intranasal Steroid Injection: indications, results, complications. *South Med J* 1978; **71**: 789.

30. Sorensen H, Mygind N, Pedersen CB, Prytz S. Long-term treatment of nasal polyps with beclomethasone dipropionate aerosol. III: Morphological studies and conclusions. *Acta Oto-laryngol (Stockholm)* 1976; **82**: 260.

31. Brogden RN, Peight TM, Avery GS. Sodium cromoglycate (cromolyn sodium). II. Allergic rhinitis and other conditions. *Drugs* 1974; **7**: 283–96.
32. Frankland AW, Walker SR. A comparison of intranasal betamethasone valerate and sodium cromoglycate in seasonal rhinitis. *Clin Allergy* 1975; **5**: 295–300.
33. Brown HM, Engler C, English JR. A comparative trial of flunisolide and sodium cromoglycate nasal sprays in the treatment of seasonal allergic rhinitis. *Clin Allergy* 1981; **11**: 169–73.
34. Illum P, Bjerrum P. Budesonide (Rhinocort) and DSCG (Lomudal) in grasspollen-induced hay-fever—a clinical comparison (abstract). *Symposium on local steroids in rhinopathies*. Lund, Sweden 1983.
35. Hillas J, Booth RJ, Somerfield S, Morton R, Avery J, Wilson JD. A comparative trial of intranasal beclomethasone dipropionate and sodium cromoglycate in patients with chronic perennial rhinitis. *Clin Allergy* 1980; **10**: 253–8.
36. Tandon MK, Strahan EG. Double-blind crossover trial comparing beclomethasone dipropionate and sodium cromoglycate in perennial allergic rhinitis. *Clin Allergy* 1980; **11**: 455–62.
37. Pegelow K-O, Gottberg L, Salomonsson P, Samuelsson A. Clinical comparison of budesonide and disodium cromoglycate in patients with hay fever (abstract). *Symposium on local steroids in rhinopathies*. Lund, Sweden 1983.
38. Harding SM, Heath S. Intranasal steroid aerosol in perennial rhinitis: comparison with an antihistamine compound *Clin Allergy* 1976; **6**: 369–72.
39. Munch EP, Soborg M, Norreslet TT, Mygind N. A comparative study of dexchlorpheniramine maleate sustained release tablets and budesonide nasal spray in seasonal allergic rhinitis. *Allergy* 1983; **38**: 517–24.

Chapter 12

THE USE OF SYSTEMIC CORTICOSTEROIDS IN THE TREATMENT OF RHINITIS

P. van Cauwenberge

Corticosteroids are highly effective in the treatment of allergic rhinitis and most cases of non-specific nasal hyperresponsiveness. Systemically administered corticosteroids would probably be the treatment of choice if they were free from side-effects. However, because of the possible serious side effects, systemic long-term treatment of rhinitis is not advisable, contrary to the situation with allergic asthma.

MECHANISMS OF ACTION

Corticosteroids have a pluripotent action on various cells. The strong antiinflammatory action influences the function of the cells, and also their migration. In addition, corticosteroids inhibit the degranulation of mast cells.

Often rhinitis does not have one single aetiology, but possesses a network of different aetiologies and sometimes one aetiology influences another. In this way an allergic reaction, as well as viral and bacterial infections of the nasal mucosa may lead to non-specific hyperresponsiveness of the mucous membranes [1, 2, 3]. It is also assumed that an allergic process in a tissue favours the establishment of infections. For these reasons it may be necessary to administer a broad spectrum treatment, e.g. corticosteroids, in severe or lingering cases of rhinitis of presumably mixed origin.

PRINCIPLES OF THERAPY

Systemic corticosteroids are preferred to topical corticosteroids or other more "conservative" treatments if a quick response is wanted or needed; the action of topical steroids is much slower [5]. In cases of severe symptoms, e.g. if the sinus ostia are involved and there is considerable oedema of the nasal mucosa causing severe headache, topical steroids and antihistamines are not active enough. In these cases a short lasting treatment (2–4 days) with orally administered corticosteroids may be very useful.

Corticosteroids are most useful when inflammatory cells are involved in the allergic process. This is, in fact, nearly always the case in allergic rhinitis, and not only in chronic disease. It has been demonstrated that in allergic rhinitis the vast majority of the cases are due to a mast cell mediated (type 1) reaction, in which mediators are released with a direct action on the cells, but also chemotactic factors, recruiting other inflammatory cells—such as neutrophils and eosinophils—to the site of allergic reaction [6]. These inflammatory cells will in turn release their own mediators and enzymes, which contribute to the chronicity of the reaction and sometimes to the appearance of a late phase reaction after a symptom free interval. In addition, degranulation of the mast cell may be caused not only by a type 1 hypersensitivity reaction, but also by many other stimuli such as viral and bacterial infection, physical and chemical irritation, stress, and many pharmacological compounds. It is, consequently, easy to understand that the three major types of rhinitis (allergic, vasomotor and infectious) have a similar symptomatology, because the input to the system is very similar although the initiating factor may be different [3].

As already mentioned, neutrophils are attracted to the site of allergic reaction by NCF, a chemotactic factor released by the mast cell. In bacterial rhinitis neutrophils are the main component of the inflammatory cells, especially in the acute phase. Eosinophils are also attracted to the site of allergic reaction by a chemotactic factor, ECFA, but can also be found in the majority of the cases of non-specific nasal hyperresponsiveness (vasomotor rhinitis). In this respect it should be emphasised that the finding of eosinophils in vasomotor rhinitis (and also in allergic rhinitis), has a prognostic value for the results of treatment, and especially of treatment with corticosteroids: patients with nasal eosinophilia respond better than patients without nasal eosinophilia.

When physicians use systemic corticosteroids in the treatment of a patient with rhinitis, they should follow some guidelines: therapy should be short-term (not more than two weeks). Whenever possible, other, less dangerous, drugs should be administered concomitantly in order to reduce the dosage of steroids. The dose should be as high as necessary but as low as needed. A thorough history taking and physical examination should be performed prior to the administration of systemic steroids, in order to detect coexisting diseases which may be a contraindication to the administration of corticosteroids.

CONTRAINDICATIONS

Contraindications for systemic steroids in rhinitis are glaucoma, herpes keratitis, chronic infection, advanced osteoporosis, severe hypertension and diabetes mellitus. Systemic steroids should not be used for rhinitis in children or during pregnancy.

PREPARATIONS

Systemic corticosteroids can be given orally (prednisolone) or as a depot injection of a micro-crystalline ester (e.g. methylprednisolone acetate).

Otorhinolaryngologists and allergists rarely use depot injections; on the other hand, general practitioners often use, and occasionally misuse, them. Their argument is that clinical experience has shown that one or two injections of a depot preparation are in nearly all instances free of serious adverse effects. However, it must be remembered that one injection of 80 mg methylprednisolone (2 ml) corresponds to 100 mg prednisolone (20 tablets of 5 mg), and that a continuous release during the day will suppress adrenal function more than a single dose given in the morning. A single injection causes a partial suppression of adrenal function, lasting for 2–3 weeks [7, 8, 9].

INDICATIONS

Seasonal allergic rhinitis

When other treatments are inadequate in hay fever, the patient can be supplied with prednisolone tablets of 5 mg [10] and instructed to take one to two tablets in the morning in periods when the symptoms are severe. The patient should, however, continue the basic therapy with antihistamines, eye drops and nasal sprays (topical steroids or cromoglycate).

Oral steroid medication has the advantage over depot injections that the treatment can be regulated according to the pollen count. In this way, unnecessary medication, e.g. during rainy periods, can be avoided. When we consider the cost-benefit ratio of the different treatments used in the treatment of seasonal allergic rhinitis, it is obvious that prednisolone is cheaper than immunotherapy, and that antihistamines are cheaper than the modern nasal sprays. According to Mygind et al. [10], the poor man's therapy for hay fever consists of antihistamine tablets during the entire season and prednisolone tablets at the peak. It is also obvious that the efforts made in the industrialised world to develop and produce drugs with an activity close to that of the best drug known for this indication, but without the side effects of it, are sensible. We should always bear in mind that rhinitis is not a life threatening disease, although it harms the quality of life. Antihistamines are most effective in itching, sneezing and rhinorrhoea, while systemic steroids, like the topical steroids, seem to be most effective on nasal blockage [11].

Perennial rhinitis and nasal polyposis

A chronic pathological condition in the nasal mucosa will respond most readily to a short term impact therapy [10]. A two-week treatment with oral corticosteroids in a patient with perennial rhinitis or nasal polyposis will often produce symptomatic relief which outlasts the pharmacological effect of the compound by one to two months.

Systemic corticosteroids can be used in this way to open up a blocked nose before topical therapy is started, or when there is a temporary failure of spray treatment, e.g. after a common cold. The value of systemic corticosteroids has, in fact, increased since the introduction of the topical steroid sprays which can maintain the effect of initial systemic steroid. The risk of adverse effects is small if there is at least three months between treatment periods [10].

Corticosteroids in perennial rhinitis and nasal polyposis can be given as a depot injection or orally, using an initially high and rapidly decreasing dose. Most arguments are in favour of the oral administration, but it can be said in favour of a depot injection that it places the treatment firmly in the hands of the physician. It ensures that the patient cannot convert what was intended as an intermittent therapy to continuous treatment, more likely to cause adverse effects by spreading out the medication [10] .

Depot injections may cause subcutaneous atrophy around the injection site. The disfiguring atrophy can last for up to two years and may not be completely reversible [12].

EFFICACY OF SYSTEMIC STEROIDS

The effect of oral steroids on rhinitis symptoms has not been studied systematically in controlled trials. In some studies it is suggested [13, 14] or demonstrated [15] that depot injections of corticosteroids have a beneficial effect in hay fever.

A recent trial performed by Borum *et al.*, with detailed symptom monitoring, has suggested that the effect of a single depot injection on nasal blockage lasts for at least four weeks, while the effect on sneezing and nose blowing is rather poor [11]. Depot injections have not been compared with other types of pharmacotherapy. One open trial suggested that one or two depot injections of corticosteroids have an effect similar to that of immunotherapy [16].

CONCLUSIONS

Systemic corticosteroids are effective in all kinds of rhinitis. Short term administration of systemic corticosteroids may be very useful when the symptoms of allergic or vasomotor rhinitis cannot be controlled by a more conservative treatment.

Because of the possible side effects of systemic corticosteroids, however, this treatment should be strictly limited to the most severe cases of rhinitis.

REFERENCES

1. Connell JT. Quantitative intranasal pollen challenges. III. The priming effect in allergic rhinitis. *J Allergy* 1969; **43**: 33–44.
2. Van Cauwenberge P, Ingels K, Declercq G. Nasal provocation with histamine in normals and in patients with allergic and non-allergic hyperreactivity. *Ann Allergy* 1985; **55**: 237.
3. Van Cauwenberge P. Sniffing out rhinitis. *J Clin Prac*, 1989 (In press).
4. Van Cauwenberge P. Infektiös-allergische Rhinosinusitis. *Allergologie (München)* 1986; **9**: 229–36.
5. Pipkorn U, Norman PS, Middleton E. Topical steroids in allergic and vasomotor

rhinitis. In: Mygind N, Weeke B, eds. *Allergic and vasomotor rhinitis.* Copenhagen: Munksgaard, 1985.

6. Van Cauwenberge P. The role of chemical mediators and neurotransmittors in rhinopathy from allergic and non-allergic origin. In: Faliaci F, ed. *Allergo-immunologia in ORL.* Roma, 1985; 26–32.

7. Ganderton MS, James VHT. Clinical and endocrine side-effects of methylprednisolone acetate as used in hay-fever. *Br Med J* 1970; **1**: 267–9.

8. Ohlander BO. A comparison of three injectable corticosteroids for the treatment of patients with seasonal hay fever. *J Int Med Res* 1980; **8**: 63–9.

9. Hedner P, Persson G. Suppression of hypothalamo-pituitary-adrenal axis after a single intramuscular injection of methylprednisolone acetate. *Ann Allergy* 1981; **47**: 176–9.

10. Mygind N, Haye R, Svedmyr N. Systemic steroids. In: Mygind N, Weeke B, eds. *Allergic and vasomotor rhinitis. Clinical aspects.* Copenhagen: Munksgaard, 1987.

11. Borum P, Gronborg H, Brofeldt S, Mygind N. Effect of a depot-injection of methylprednisolone in hay fever (In preparation, cited by Mygind *et al.*, 1987).

12. Haye R, Kolbenstvedt A. Local atrophy at the site of injection of depot steroids. *Tidsskr Nor Lageforen* 1984; **104**: 1532–3.

13. Chervinsky P. Treatment of seasonal allergic rhinitis with long-acting steroid injections. A comparison of four preparations. *Ann Allergy* 1968; **26**: 190–3.

14. Kronholm A. Injectable depot corticosteroid therapy in hay fever. *J Int Med Res* 1979; **7**: 314–7.

15. Brown E, Seideman T, Seigelaub AB, Popovitz C. Depot-methylprednisolone in the treatment of ragweed hayfever. *Ann Allergy* 1960; **18** : 1321–30.

16. Ganderton MA, Brostoff J, Frankland AW. Comparison of preseasonal and coseasonal Allpyral with Depo-Medrone in summer hay-fever. *Br Med J* 1969; **1**: 357–8.

Chapter 13

SURGERY IN ALLERGIC AND VASOMOTOR RHINITIS

A. F. van Olphen

INTRODUCTION

Allergic rhinitis is caused by an immunological response, whereas vasomotor rhinitis is a result of an imbalance in the autonomic nervous system [1]. The main symptoms of both conditions are attacks of paroxysmal sneezing, nasal obstruction and copious watery rhinorrhoea. In some instances there may in addition be conjunctival irritation with increased lacrimation.

Regarding the aetiology it is obvious that surgery is not the treatment of first choice. Nevertheless there are indications for surgery in these conditions. The aims of surgery are to correct anatomical abnormalities, to reduce swelling by introducing scar tissue and by destroying blood vessels, to remove irreversibly diseased tissues such as polyps, and to interrupt the parasympathetic innervation of the nose. For these purposes functional corrective nasal surgery, turbinate surgery, polypectomy, sinus surgery and surgery of the parasympathetic nervous system are available.

FUNCTIONAL CORRECTIVE NASAL SURGERY

Functional corrective nasal surgery has been developed to improve the physiology of the nose by correction of the septum and the external pyramid. It is often indicated in allergic and vasomotor rhinitis, not only for its direct effect on the nasal patency, but also for an indirect effect on the degree of filling of the submucosal vascular plexus by a reflex mechanism as postulated by Graamans [2].

Examination of the septum can be conducted with a speculum and adequate illumination. The most frequent findings are deviations,

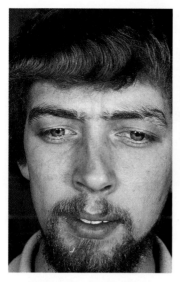
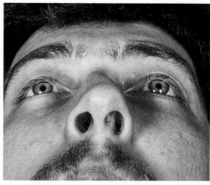

Figure 1: Deviated cartilaginous dorsum and luxation of caudal septum. Restoration of the nasal function requires correction of both the internal and the external nose.

spurs and spines. However inspection of the vestibule and valve should be made without a speculum, because its blades may cover the skin of the vestibule or disturb the valve by moving the ala in a lateral position. Special attention should be given to the valve area. This is the narrowest part of the respiratory tract. For this reason minor abnormalities have a great impact. Consequently even minor improvements in the valve area can result in a considerable relief of complaints.

From a functional point of view deviated pyramids, prominent narrow noses and weak lobules deserve attention. A deviation in the external pyramid often impedes correction of a deformity in the septum (Fig.1). A prominent nose results in a slot shaped breathing surface in the internal and external ostium. By lowering the nose these ostia will be widened, resulting in a larger breathing surface. A weak lobule will collapse during inspiration due to the Venturi effect. The result is a strong increase in inspiratory nasal resistance. It is most difficult to correct this abnormality. The foregoing demonstrates that in order to achieve a normal physiology of the nose attention should be paid to both the internal and external nose.

Gustav Kilian (1860–1921) [3, 4] and Otto Tiger Freer (1857–1932) [5, 6] promoted the submucosal resection of the septum. This was the first useful treatment of septal deformities. The disadvantages of the submucosal resection are that there is a great risk of perforations of the septum, sagging of the dorsum and retraction of the columella. In order to prevent the latter two, a strut of cartilage has to be preserved in the dorsum and columella, making it impossible to correct deformities in these areas.

Nowadays the treatment of choice is the functional and corrective nasal surgery which was promoted by Maurice H. Cottle (1898–1981) [7, 8] . In functional and corrective nasal surgery all areas of the septum can be corrected. Only superfluous cartilage and bone is removed. If necessary deformed parts of the septum are resected and later on reconstructed by implantation. This results in an optimal support of the nasal dorsum and the columella after surgery and it prevents septal perforations. Various corrections of the pyramid can be made by osteotomies, resections and implantation. The septum forms the medial support of the pyramid. An immobile septum will keep the pyramid in place. Therefore a pyramid correction should always be made in combination with a septum correction.

TURBINATE SURGERY

Zuckerkandl [9] pointed out that there is a large variety in the form of the turbinates. The size of the turbinates depends on the dimensions of their skeleton and the filling of the submucus vascular plexuses. The superior turbinate is frequently absent [10, 11]. The middle turbinate sometimes contains a large aerated sinus, which can be seen as a continuation of the ethmoidal sinus.

The turbinate plays an important role in the physiology of the nose. Its presence results in turbulent airflow and in a large surface area of mucous membranes, which facilitates warming and humidifying of the air. Furthermore the turbulent flow brings inhaled small particles into contact with the mucus on the membranes. These particles stick to the mucus and will be transported by the mucociliary movement to the nasopharynx. The submucosal vascular plexus is part of a system regulating the nasal resistance.

In order to see if there is an enlargement based on the size of the skeleton or swelling of the mucous membranes, examination of the turbinates should always be done before and after decongestion. Regular observations are: an enlarged skeleton, which makes a septum correction impossible (Fig.2); obstruction of the ostia of the sinuses; swelling; hypertrophy; and polypoid degeneration. There

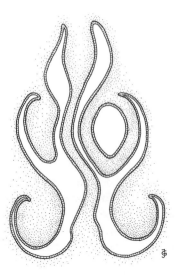

Figure 2: Bullous medial turbinate. Surgery of the bullous turbinate is necessary to facilitate a septum correction.

are various surgical procedures to correct these. However, one should keep in mind that too vigorous surgery may result in atrophic rhinitis, a disease characterised by crust formation and atrophy of the mucous membranes. The main symptoms are headache, blockage of the nose and fetor. The fetor can ruin one's social life! Atrophic rhinitis is very hard to cure; consequently it should be prevented at all costs. Nevertheless surgery is frequently indicated. The aims of turbinate surgery are to reduce swelling, to remove polypoid degenerated tissue and to reduce the size of the turbinate.

Various caustic procedures have been used to reduce swelling by destroying the submucosal tissues, especially the blood vessels, and promoting the formation of scar tissue. For this purpose chemical agents, electrocoagulation, diathermy and cryosurgery are available. In general these procedures have an initially beneficial effect, but long term results are disappointing. Another disadvantage of these techniques is that the mucous membranes are severed at the risk of an atrophic rhinitis. In my view only bipolar submucosal diathermy can be advocated, since this technique leaves the mucous membranes intact, but it should be restricted to selected cases. Generally surgical removal of redundant soft tissues gives a better and long lasting result and it is less destructive.

Correction of the skeleton of the turbinates is more complicated. It requires a submucosal approach, which makes it possible to perform all kinds of corrections without damaging the soft tissues, eg reducing a bullous middle turbinate, by resection of one wall of the bulla and reducing a spongiform middle or lower turbinate by compression and trimming [12].

POLYPECTOMY

Changes in the mucous membranes and polyp formation disturb the mucociliary clearance. They also block the nose and the ostia of the sinuses. This gives rise to an increased susceptibility to infections. Once the tissues are irreversibly changed or polyps are present surgery is the most effective solution. Polyps are a major problem in rhinology. Even after careful polypectomy there is a strong tendency to recurrences. Local steroids can be used to try and prevent this [13, 14]. Sometimes even small polyps require treatment, because they can, depending on their location, cause obstruction of the ostia of the sinuses. More about polyps can be found in Chapter 9.

SINUS SURGERY

Most infections of the nose and paranasal sinuses are self limiting diseases and do not require treatment other than for relief of symptoms. However, infections in allergic rhinitis have a tendency to last longer than normal or to become chronic. In order to prevent this, it is advisable to take simple measures during infections to prevent stasis of discharges in the nose. For this purpose washouts of the nose with saline can be helpful. In more severe cases antibiotics can be given in combination with decongestants like xylometazoline. However, one should bear in mind that, especially in allergic patients, xylometazoline might lead to addiction. If the treatment as described above is unsuccessful, sinus washouts are indicated. When the condition does not respond to conservative treatment surgery has to be performed.

The aim of surgery is to improve drainage of the sinuses and to remove irreversibly diseased tissue. Preoperative examinations consist of X-ray photography, ultrasonic scanning of the sinuses, and endoscopy. The first gives information about all sinuses, ultrasonic scanning only about the maxillary and frontal sinuses and endoscopy only about the nasal cavity and the maxillary sinus. Of these examinations, endoscopy reveals the most detailed information about the patency of the ostia, the mucociliary movement, polyp formation, cysts and the condition of the mucous membranes.

Transnasal ethmoidectomy is frequently performed to remove polyps and to improve drainage from the ethmoidal, the maxillary and frontal sinuses. If only drainage is required infundibulotomy can be performed [15]. The introduction of endoscopic and microsurgical techniques contributed very much to the development and propagation of these surgical procedures [16]. With these the risks of serious complications like blindness and liquorrhoea are reduced to an acceptable level. It is then possible, with extreme care, to make drainage openings from the ethmoidal and maxillary sinus to the nose. These openings are in the best position with regard to mucociliary movement, giving optimal clearance of the sinuses. Transantral ethmoidectomy is only done when pathology in the maxillary sinus requires a Caldwell-Luc operation or when effective surgery or safety requires a better view into the ethmoidal sinus.

The classic antrostomy according to Claoué is made in the medial wall of the sinus under the inferior turbinate. Properly made it gives a good ventilation of the sinus. However taking the mucociliary movement into account it is not the preferred side. The Caldwell-Luc operation gives access to the antrum through a labiogingival incision and opening of the anterior wall of the sinus. This operation is the best way to remove polyps, cysts and irreversibly diseased mucous membranes. Originally the antrostoma in this operation is made under the inferior turbinate. Some surgeons prefer a more physiological side as described previously. During a Caldwell-Luc operation a transantral ethmoidectomy can be done. This approach gives a wide access to the ethmoidal sinus, which enables an operation without the help of advanced endoscopic and microsurgical techniques. However there is a high rate of postoperative algesia and hypaesthesia. The diseases for which a Caldwell-Luc operation is indicated have a high rate of recurrence. Therefore this operation should be reserved for cases where there is no other solution.

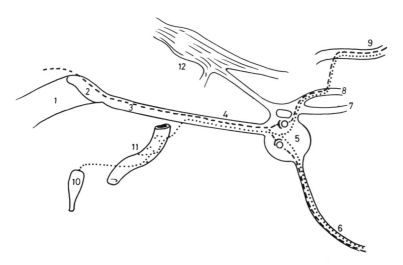

Figure 3: The autonomic innervation of the nose. 1,Facial Nerve; 2,Geniculate ganglion; 3,Greater petrosal nerve; 4,Nerve of the pterygoid canal (vidian nerve); 5,Pterygopalatine ganglion; 6,Nasopalatine nerve; 7,Maxillary nerve; 8,Zygomatic nerve; 9,Lacrimal nerve; 10,Superior cervical ganglion; 11,Internal carotid artery.

SURGERY OF THE PARASYMPATHETIC NERVOUS SYSTEM

Parasympathetic fibres from the facial nerve reach the pterygopalatine ganglion through the greater petrosal nerve and the nerve of the pterygoid canal (vidian nerve). The post ganglionic fibres pass through the nasopalatine nerve to the glands in the nasal mucous membranes and through the maxillary, zygomatic and lacrimal nerve to the lacrimal glands (Fig.3). Stimulation of these parasympathetic fibres activates nasal secretion.

Malcolmson [17] introduced the resection of nerve of the pterygoid canal in the pterygopalatine fossa near the pterygopalatine ganglion. This method was promoted by Golding-Wood [18]. The pterygoid fossa is opened via a transantral approach, which might lead to postoperative algesia and hypaesthesia as mentioned before. Another side effect is conjunctival irritation by insufficient lacrimation.

There is, however, a simpler way to interrupt the parasympathetic innervation of the nose, which makes use of the fact that the nasopalatine nerve can be reached relatively easily at the sphenopalatine foramen, where it enters the nasal cavity. This foramen is situated in the lateral wall of the nasal cavity posterior to the medial turbinate and close to the sphenoid sinus. Coagulation of the nerve at this spot can be relatively easily performed as an office procedure, avoiding the disadvantages of a transantral approach of the pterygopalatine fossa and impaired lacrimation.

Although good results of these operations have been reported, long term results were unsatisfactory [19]. The most likely explanation for this is reinnervation. Therefore an operation as invasive as the transantral neurectomy is not justified. The transnasal coagulation of the nasopalatine nerve at the sphenopalatine foramen can be helpful to achieve a short term relief of symptoms. Since this operation is not very invasive a second operation can be considered after recurrence of symptoms.

REFERENCES

1. Änggard A. Vasomotor rhinitis-pathophysiological aspects. *Rhinology* 1979; **17**: 31-5.
2. Graamans K. Does septal surgery influence submucous congestion? *Rhinology* 1983; **21**: 21-7.
3. Kilian G. *Einleitung Zur Diskusion über die operative Therapie der Septumdeviation*. Verhandl. Gesellschaft Deut. Naturforscher u. ˙Arzte. Vogel, Liepzig 1899; 392-393.
4. Kilian G. Die submuköse Fensterresektion der Nasenscheidewand. *Arch Laryng Rhinol* 1904; **16**: 362-87.
5. Freer OT. The correction of deflections of the nasal septum with minimum of traumatism. JAMA 1902; **38**: 636-42.
6. Freer OT. Deflections of the septum. *Ann Otol* 1905; **14** : 213-66.
7. Cottle MH. *Corrective surgery on nasal septum and external pyramid*. Chicago: Am Rhin Soc, 1960.
8. *The collected writings of Maurice H Cottle, M.D.* Editorial Board, Pat A. Barelli, Walter E.E. Loch, Eugene B. Kern and Albert Steiner. Chicago: Am Rhin Soc, 1987.
9. Zuckerkandl E. *Normale und pathologische Anatomie der ʾNasenhöhle und ihrer pneumatischen Anhänge, 2*. Aufl., Bd. I. Braumüller, Wien 1893; 368-400.11
10. Lange J. *Klinische Anatomie der Nase, Nasenhöhle und Nebenhöhlen*. Stuttgart/New York: Georg Thieme Verlag, 1988.
11. Messerklinger, W. III Die Endoskopie der Nase und der Nebenhöhlen. In: Berendes J, Link R, Zöllner F. *Hals-Nasen- und ohrenheilkunde in Praxis und Klinik*. Stuttgart/New York: Georg Thieme Verlag, 1977.
12. Pirsig W. Reduction of the middle turbinate. *Rhinol* 1972; **10**: 103-8.
13. Virolainen E, Puhakka H. The effect of intranasal beclomethasone dipropionate on the recurrence of nasal polyps after ethmoidectomy. *Rhinology* 1980; **18**: 9-18.
14. Drettner B, Ebbesen A, Nilsson M. Prophylactic treatment with flunisolide after polypectomy. *Rhinology* 1982; **20**: 149-58.
15. Messerklinger W. Das Infundibulum ethmoidale und seine entzündlichen Erkrankungen. *Arch. ORL* 1979; **222**: 11-22.
16. Wigand ME. Transnasal ethmoidectomy under endoscopical control. *Rhinology* 1981; **19**: 7-15.

17. Malcolmson KG. The vasomotor activities of the nasal mucous membrane. *J Laryngol Otol* 1959; **73**: 73-98.
18. Golding-Wood PH. Pathology and surgery of chronic vasomotor rhinitis. *J Laryngol* 1962; **76**: 969-77.
19. Krant JN, *et al.* Long-term results of vidian neurectomy. *Rhinology* 1979; **17**: 231-5.

Chapter 14

NASAL ALLERGY IN CHILDREN

J. O. Warner

INTRODUCTION

Allergic rhinitis is a very common chronic disorder, occurring in approximately 10% of children and up to 20% of adolescents and young adults [1]. It occurs in 75% of children with asthma which itself is a very common condition [2]. However, it is frequently undiagnosed and its importance as a cause of morbidity underestimated. It has a profound effect on school performance and in this respect under-achievment at examinations which are often inappropriately held during the height of the pollen season is common. Seasonal allergic rhinitis is estimated to occur in between 5% and 9% of children but is quite rare under the age of five. Isolated perennial rhinitis occurs in around 3% of children but in association with perennial asthma is infinitely more common [2].

CLINICAL FEATURES

Symptoms may be perennial, seasonal, or provoked by specific precipitants. Seasonal and specific allergy-provoked symptoms tend to be more acute, severe, and more likely to be associated with conjunctivitis by comparison with perennial rhinitis. Symptoms include nasal congestion (stuffy nose), sneezing, itching, and rhinorrhoea. The latter may be associated with either a clear or creamy nasal discharge. It may be possible to elicit information on specific precipitants from the history such as exposure to animal danders. However, many children with allergic rhinitis have symptoms triggered by non-specific irritants such as cigarette smoke, strong paint fumes or odours, as well as by exposure to allergens. Noisy oro-nasal breathing, a nasal voice and snoring may also be reported. Older children may note loss of smell (an- or hypo-osmia) and this may lead to a loss of appetite. Repeated throat

215

clearing and coughing especially at night may also be noted. The noisy breathing, irritating sniffing, coughing and throat clearing often lead to social isolation at school and discord at home. General symptoms such as nausea, headaches, fatigue, irritability and poor concentration may also occur. Itching of the pharynx and palate, hearing loss and popping of the ears with earache may be reported by older patients. Patients with associated conjunctivitis complain of sore, red, itchy and runny eyes.

Timing of symptoms will provide the most useful guide to specific allergy diagnosis. Knowledge of tree, grass pollen and mould spore counts will help delineate specific allergies which can then be confirmed by appropriate investigation. The most common cause of perennial symptoms is an allergy to house dust mite and here a history of profuse sneezing on arising in the morning with progressive improvement of symptoms during the day is typical. Symptoms may also be associated with domestic activities such as bed making and vacuum cleaning. In children bouncing on the bed and pillow fights may be more likely triggers.

Many patients will have had or still have associated atopic disorders such as bronchial asthma, atopic dermatitis, gastrointestinal food intolerances, urticaria and angio-oedema. Likewise similar symptoms may have been present in first degree relatives. Additional questioning will be required to distinguish non-allergic causes of rhinitis. These will be discussed in the section on differential diagnosis.

CLINICAL EXAMINATION

Children with nasal allergy often develop characteristic mannerisms such as nose wrinkling and twitching. Many repeatedly rub the tip of their nose with the dorsum of the hand which is the characteristic so-called "allergic salute". This will eventually result in a transverse crease just below the bridge of the nose. Dark rings are often apparent under the eyes with some puffiness of the peri-orbital skin. This is attributed to venous stasis due to impaired blood flow through the swollen nasal mucosa. The appearance is often known as "the allergic shiners". The nasal bridge may be broadened secondary to chronic nasal obstruction and will be particularly apparent if there are nasal polyps present.

Examination of the lower third of nasal cavity is easily performed using an auroscope though visualisation will be enhanced by the use of a nasal speculum with illumination from a head light or head mirror. The nasal mucosa usually appears oedematous and congested. Whilst a pale or violaceous appearance is usually associated with allergic rhinitis, this is not always present. Watery mucoid or opaque material may be noted in the nasal cavities and posterior pharyngeal wall. Blood crusting in Little's area may be a feature of the condition, particularly in children who continually pick their nose.

Children with chronic nasal obstruction and mouth breathing often have halitosis, though this is more particularly a feature of foreign body in the nose or anatomical obstruction due to incomplete choanal atresia. Orthodontic anomalies may also be a consequence of mouth breathing. Examination of the ears is essential in all children. Retracted tympanic membranes and signs of fluid in the middle ears is common. At least 20% of children with allergic rhinitis have middle ear abnormalities [3]. Hearing deficits are also common and it is particularly important that these should be detected and treated to avoid the inevitable learning difficulties and speech defects which ensue. In patients with associated conjunctivitis the bulbar conjunctiva shows hyperaemia and thickening. At its most severe vernal seasonal conjunctivitis leads to a cobblestone appearance of the tarsal conjunctiva with itching, redness of the eye, lacrimation and a mucinous discharge. During active disease small erosions develop in the cornea which lead to photophobia and ptosis. At its most severe corneal ulcerations may also occur.

Full physical examination may reveal signs of past or present atopic dermatitis, such as skin pigmentation, depigmentation and chronic lichenification, particularly around skin flexures. Thoracic cage deformity with bowing of the sternum and Harrison sulci will indicate the presence of obstructive airways disease and auscultation may reveal polyphonic expiratory wheezing characteristic of asthma.

DIFFERENTIAL DIAGNOSIS

Vasomotor rhinitis

Non-infectious non-allergic rhinitis is relatively uncommon in childhood. Symptoms are intermittent and perennial and may be provoked by changes in environmental temperature or exposure to irritants.

Foreign body in the nasal cavity

Rhinitis secondary to foreign body should be suspected in children with a unilateral foul smelling or bloody nasal discharge with extremely unpleasant halitosis. Young children are particularly prone to inserting objects into their nose and it may be some weeks or even months before this becomes apparent due to secondary infection.

Chronic infective rhinitis

Mucopurulent rhinorrhoea which may be associated in older children with sinusitis and in younger children with purulent otitis media in addition to repeated lower respiratory tract infection may be a feature of a number of generalised disorders.

Cystic fibrosis Cystic fibrosis pre-disposes to chronic infection in the nose and sinuses as well as in the lung. Nasal polyps occur in up to 20% of children with this condition. Indeed, any children with nasal polyps should have a mandatory sweat test to exclude this diagnosis. Usually the nasal symptoms will be associated with other more typical features of cystic fibrosis, namely recurrent and chronic chest infections and failure to thrive, with steatorrhoea due to pancreatic insufficiency. However, a small percentage of patients with cystic fibrosis present with recurrent nasal polyps and appear to have otherwise relatively mild disease. The condition is autosomal, recessively inherited and diagnosed by the finding of a raised sodium and chloride content of the sweat [4].

Ciliary dyskinesia syndrome Fifty per cent of patients with this condition have dextrocardia and situs inversus. It is associated with chronic upper and lower respiratory tract infection with the ultimate development of bronchiectasis. The most characteristic feature in the clinical history is a neonatal onset of upper and lower respiratory tract symptoms [5]. It is diagnosed by the finding of decreased nasal clearance rates, abnormalities of ciliary beat frequency and ultrastructural abnormalities of the cilia.

Immune deficiency Chronic infections in the nose and sinuses may be a feature of an underlying immune deficiency such as hypogammaglobulinaemia. However, this is likely to be associated with recurrent infections elsewhere.

Mechanical obstruction Hypertrophy of lymphoid tissue in the adenoids and tonsils may produce marked nasal obstruction with secondary infection. Deviated nasal septum will produce a similar problem. Much rarer are congenital anomalies such as incomplete choanal atresia, encephalocoele or meningocoele which may produce nasal obstruction.

Granulomatous disorders such as Wegener's granulomatosis and sarcoidosis are extremely rare in childhood but may produce nasal obstruction.

INVESTIGATIONS

It is usually not possible to examine the nasopharynx with mirrors in a small child and fibreoptic rhinoscopy would require heavy sedation and local anaesthetic. An X-ray of the post-nasal space will easily demonstrate adenoidal hypertrophy as a cause for nasal obstruction. Nasal secretions can be aspirated to examine for the presence of eosinophils which would support a diagnosis of allergy compared with neutrophils which would be found in infective rhinitis. Allergy prick skin tests can be easily performed in children of all ages to support the diagnosis of allergic rhinitis; 90% of atopic individuals would be identified by merely using a positive and negative control with house dust mite (*Dermatophagoides pteronyssinus*), cat fur and grass pollen. There is no contra-indication to performing skin tests even on small infants though the positive yield is less than in older children. The measurement of serum total IgE level can be particularly useful in small children to identify the presence of atopy and even predict its development. Levels of greater than 1 IU/ml at birth and 10 at one year of age are highly predictive. Specific IgE antibodies may be identified by various techniques such as the radioallergosorbent technique (RAST) or a chemiluminescent assay. Both skin tests and IgE antibody tests should be used to confirm the clinical history but should not be used in place of the history as a screen for allergic disease. The correlation between such tests and nasal challenge is good for seasonal allergens but sometimes misleading for perennial allergens such as the house dust mite. If food allergy is genuinely involved this can usually only be identified by elimination, diet and challenge.

Intra-nasal challenge can be performed in small children. Anterior rhinomanometry to detect changes in resistance can be used in children down to the age of four. Posterior rhinomanometry and peak nasal inspiratory flow requires more patient cooperation and is usually only reproduceable beyond the age of 6 or 7. Nasal challenges are usually only a research tool. Utilising this technique is has been possible to demonstrate late allergic responses. In a study of nasal provocation in atopic children symptomatic allergic rhinitis was strongly associated with late rather than immediate nasal reactions [6].

THE ORIGINS OF ALLERGY

Allergy is probably the commonest manifestation of immunodeficiency. It occurs in 15–20% of the population and amounts to one third of all chronic disease of childhood. The immunological abnormalities most commonly associated with allergy include the opsonisation defect, immunoglobulin A deficiency, immunoglobulin G subclass II deficiency and a low second component of complement level. Allergy also occurs more frequently in patients with cystic fibrosis. Such primary defects appear to influence the incidence of the allergic status but not necessarily of allergic disease. Environmental influences play an important role in influencing the manifestations of allergy. Factors such as month of birth, infant feeding practices, sex, age and intercurrent viral infections are probably important. As the immune system is particularly susceptible to sensitisation in early infancy, perhaps because of transient anomalies of immune response, allergen load in the first few months of life may be particularly important. Thus, being born just before or during the pollen season considerably increases the probability of having pollen allergy. Exposure to high concentrations of house mite which may be influenced by month of birth and type of housing is also important. Viral infection and possibly also cigarette smoke exposure adjuvantises the sensitisation process. These observations suggest that some allergic disease may be preventable by appropriate manipulation of the environment particularly in early infancy. Thus, breast feeding, avoidance of passive cigarette smoke exposure, appropriate housing with low house dust mite exposure and not being exposed to animal danders in infancy may all be of value [7]. The organ in which allergy is manifest is under additional influences, many of which may be genetic. There is an HLA antigen linkage with particular manifestations. Thus, the HLA antigen combination A3-B7 is more likely to be associated with hay fever than the combination A1 and B8 which is more commonly associated with eczema [8].

MANAGEMENT

The treatment of allergic rhinitis will be divided into avoidance of provoking factors, pharmacotherapy and in very selected instances immunotherapy or hyposensitisation as it is sometimes known.

Avoidance of provoking factors

Parents of children with allergic rhinitis should always be told to avoid smoking tobacco in front of their children. Avoidance of other non-specific factors such as paint fumes, dust, and exhaust fumes will also reduce symptoms. Unfortunately, house dust mite avoidance in homes that already have very high concentrations of house mite have been very disappointing. Modern energy saving devices such as draught exclusion and double glazing have merely served to increase humidity and decrease air exchanges within the home which enhances the proliferation of house mites. Damp housing has a similar effect. As one of the major exposures occurs in the bedroom, attention to the bed may have beneficial effects. Removal of soft toys, the use of synthetic rather than feather filled pillows and duvets and regular vacuuming of the mattress will all reduce house mite levels. Vinyl flooring rather than carpeting may also help. There are a number of anti-mite sprays on the market but currently there are none of proven efficacy. Removal of offending pets from the home must be recommended though it may take several months for the dander to be completely cleared from the dust. Appropriate air conditioning and filters may reduce indoor pollen and mould counts and be associated with a reduction in symptoms [9].

Ingestion of hot and spicy foods may exacerbate pre-existing allergic rhinitis. However, food intolerance as a cause of this condition is rare. There is very little evidence that milk or indeed any other food is a particularly common cause of rhinitis. Thus, exclusion diets are usually not indicated. Where history suggests that food may be involved, diet and challenge may be indicated [10].

PHARMACOTHERAPY

There are four main classes of drugs which may be used in rhinitis: adrenergic and anticholinergic drugs; antihistamines; sodium cromoglycate, and topical corticosteroids.

Adrenergic drugs administered topically will produce vasoconstriction and reduce oedema of the nasal mucosa. They can produce immediate relief in nasal blockage but are not indicated for allergic rhinitis. Indeed, continued use may produce troublesome side effects including hyperactive behaviour, tremor, insomnia and atrophic rhinitis. Anticholinergic drugs may be of value. Ipratropium bromide is a particularly safe product which can reduce nasal discharge significantly [11].

Antihistamines still form the mainstay of treatment of allergic rhinitis in children. The new generation of nonsedative specific H_1 receptor antagonists should now be used. There is a wide range of these new antihistamines including terfenadine, astemizole, loratadine and cetirizine. They all are associated with a very low incidence of sedation with a high-potency antihistamine effect. Many younger children with allergic rhinitis can be controlled on these antihistamines alone. Adult doses may be used even in small children. It is preferable to use them prophylactically rather than awaiting the development of symptoms, particularly in seasonal rhinitis. Used long term, these antihistamines may even have a small anti-asthma effect [12].

Sodium cromoglycate is an exclusively topically active anti-allergy compound. Its exact mode of action is still not elucidated but it can prevent both early and late allergen induced responses in the nose. Its duration of action is only four hours and in clinical practice it must be used prophylactically on a regular basis at least three and up to six times per day. Whilst double blind trials have demonstrated the efficacy of this compound compared with placebo the dose frequency required for satisfactory effect is difficult to maintain. Nevertheless its lack of toxicity and incredible safety record over 20 years of use suggests that it is a treatment that should be tried [13].

Topically active glucocorticoids with a low systemic activity are highly efficacious in the treatment of both seasonal and perennial allergic rhinitis. They decrease obstruction to a far greater extent than rhinorrhoea and sneezing. They are effective even when administered only twice daily and have a very good safety record over 15 years of use. The two compounds most widely used in the UK are beclomethasone dipropionate and budesonide. The dosage of these agents is identical in children and adults. However, children need to be taught very carefully how to use the drugs correctly and require regular monitoring of their inhalation technique.

The dose of nasal corticosteroid should be kept to the minimum required to control symptoms as even low doses can have a systemic effect. When added to inhaled corticosteroid for asthma, the total dose from the two routes of administration may be excessive. Growth suppression has been noted with total daily doses as low as $600\mu g$ per day [14].

IMMUNOTHERAPY

Immunotherapy consists of slowly increasing doses of allergen administered sequentially to allergic patients in an attempt to reduce their sensitivity to the allergen. The optimal dose, dose interval and duration of therapy are chosen arbitrarily. The administration is usually by subcutaneous injection, though there have been advocates of nasal, bronchial and oral routes. Adverse reactions still occasionally result in death following the use, or more frequently the misuse, of the treatment. Its administration is time-consuming, inconvenient and expensive. Thus, it is not a first line treatment for allergic rhinitis. However, in patients poorly controlled on optimal environmental manipulation and pharmacotherapy, immuno-therapy may be considered. Its value has been most satisfactorily proven in patients with seasonal allergic rhinitis. Pollen immunisation for one or more years has been associated with significant clinical improvement and reductions in requirements for other therapy. House dust mite immunotherapy has also been proved to be of greater benefit than placebo injections but perennial house mite- induced allergic rhinitis is usually adequately controlled with pharmacotherapy [15].

COMPARATIVE STUDIES OF THERAPIES

Inhaled corticosteroids have been found to be superior to sodium cromoglycate and antihistamines for the relief of allergic rhinitis though they tend to relieve nasal obstruction rather more than sneezing and rhinorrhoea. Antihistamines and ocular sodium cromoglycate are most appropriate for conjunctivitis. The combination of inhaled beclomethasone dipropionate and ingested H_1 specific histamine antagonists have been shown to be the best combination for long-term therapy of allergic rhinitis [12].

REFERENCES

1. Smith J M. The epidemiology of allergic rhinitis. In: Settipane G A, ed. *Rhinitis*. Providence, Rhode Island, New England and Regional Allergy Proceedings, 1984; 86–91.
2. Viner A S, Jackman N. Retrospective survey of 1271 patients diagnosed as perennial rhinitis. *Clin Allergy* 1976; **6**: 251–9.
3. Bernstein J M, Ellis E, LI P. The role of IgE-mediated hypersensitivity in otitis media with effusion. *Otolaryngol Head Neck Surg* 1981; **89**: 874–8.
4. Hodson M E, Norman A P, Batten J C. *Cystic fibrosis*. London: Baillière Tindall, 1983.
5. Buchdahl R M, Reiser J, Ingram D, Rutman A, Cole P J, Warner J O. Ciliary abnormalities in respiratory disease. *Arch Dis Childh* 1988; **63**: 238–43.
6. Price J F, Hey E N, Soothill J F. Antigen provocation to the skin, nose, and lung in children with asthma; immediate and dual hypersensitivity reactions. *Clin Exp Immunol* 1982; **47**: 587.
7. Warner J O. Allergies in childhood. In: Macfarlane J A, ed.*Progress in child health* Vol 2. Edinburgh: Churchill Livingstone, 1985; 63–76.
8. Turner M W, Brostoff J, Wells R S, Stokes C R, Soothill J F. HLA in eczema and hay fever. *Clin Exp Immunol* 1977; **27**: 43.
9. Warner J O, Boner A L. Allergy and childhood asthma. *Clin Immunol Allergy* 1988; **2**: 217–29.
10. Wraith D G, Merrett J, Roth A, Wyman L, Merrett T G. Recognition of food allergic patients and their allergens by the RAST technique and clinical investigation. *Clin Allergy* 1979; **9**: 25–36.
11. Borum P, Larsen F S, Mygind M. Intranasal ipratropium: a new treatment for perennial rhinitis. *Clin Otolaryngol* 1979; **4**: 47.
12. Simons F E R. Allergic Rhinitis: Recent Advances. *Pediatr Clin N Am* 1988; **35**: 1053–74.
13. Church M K, Warner J O. Sodium cromoglycate and related drugs. *Clin Allergy* 1985; **15**: 311–20.
14. Law C M, Marchant J L, Honour J W, Preece M A, Warner J O. Nocturnal adrenal suppression in asthmatic children taking inhaled beclomethasone dipropionate. *Lancet* 1986; **i**: 942–4.
15. Warner J O. Immunotherapy. In: Lessof M H, ed. *Allergy: Immunological and clinical aspects*. Chichester: Wiley, 1984; 447– 64.

Chapter 15

ALLERGIC CONDITIONS OF THE NOSE IN ASTHMATIC PATIENTS

G. Boyd

Epidemiological studies indicate that between 10–15% of the population develop symptoms of allergic bronchial asthma at some time during their lives. The likelihood of this occurring is much higher in the younger age group, particularly in children of early school age. This ability to mount an allergic response mediated by IgE mechanisms following contact with agents to which the individual has become sensitised results in allergic manifestations which relate to the site of entry or contact with the particular offending material. Thus inhalation of allergen can produce allergic problems in the upper airways with irritation of the nasal mucosa in addition to involvement of the lower respiratory tract and allergic bronchial asthma. Allergen contact with the eyes will result in conjunctivitis and skin contact can produce acute urticarial responses. Ingestion of allergen produces a more complex picture often with involvement of all these sites to a varying degree.

The basic function of both the upper and the lower airways is to warm and humidify inspired air and to conduct it to the lower gas exchanging parts of the lung. Although they share common functions, the upper and lower airways have different structures so that their inherent responses to contact with inhaled allergen will produce different reactions.

The nasal mucosa is likely to be subjected to a greater allergen load than the bronchial surface but allergic manifestations, although reflecting the different anatomical and histological structure of the nasal mucosa as compared to the bronchial mucosa, tend to parallel each other at these different sites. The reaction which occurs in the nasal mucosa is more susceptible to antihistamine administration and not beta$_2$ agonists; a situation which is reversed at the bronchial site. Steroid preparations, however, suppress the allergic reaction effectively in all areas.

It is well recognised that although 10–15% of the population are atopic, i.e. have the capacity to mount an IgE mediated allergic reaction, not all of these individuals do so and, indeed, the level of allergic reactivity will vary throughout life so that, at times, the level of allergic responsiveness is high and symptoms of asthma or rhinitis are prominent, whereas at other times, when the level of allergic responsiveness is low, the individual can be symptomatic. There is a close interaction between the different parts of the airways in relation to the level of allergic reactivity. A patient with pollen induced seasonal allergic rhinitis therefore can present initially with nasal symptoms alone when the antigenic stimulus first appears, and as the antigen load increases, the level of reactivity also rises with more prominent symptoms and the development of increasing bronchial hyperreactivity with the emergence of bronchospasm. In a highly susceptible individual, minor irritation in the upper airways, such as exposure to certain fumes or scents, can precipitate an acute bronchial response together with symptoms of asthma.

Allergic conditions in the nose cause seasonal and/or perennial rhinitis and will affect some 15–20% of the population. The fact that 10% have perennial symptoms underlines the likelihood of nasal symptoms being associated closely with respiratory allergic responses. Overall it would appear that about 50% of those who suffer from perennial rhinitis are atopic with evidence of positive IgE mediated skin responses and hypersensitivity to the house dust mite is implicated in the majority of these. This figure is much higher in children where some 80% with nasal symptoms are atopic and it falls to around 20% in those over 60 years of age. Nasal allergy is common, particularly in children and although it can occur readily by itself, some 85% of those who present with bronchial asthma have evidence of an allergic rhinitis in addition. It is always relevant, therefore, to examine the nose for evidence of an allergic mucosal reaction in any child who presents with recurring chest problems associated with cough with or without wheeze.

Allergic conditions within the nose present with symptoms of nasal discharge, nasal blockage, sneezing and irritation although the severity of each will vary in different individuals. Other problems associated with itchiness of the eyes, throat and ears occur commonly and reduced sense of smell is a frequent finding although this is not always readily elicited in children. Rhinitis is not a life threatening condition but is always debilitating and significantly reduces the quality of life. Most individuals are unaware that it can be treated and most of those with asthma are much more concerned with control of their bronchospasm and alleviation of their respiratory symptoms so that they will tolerate the nasal problem frequently without comment or complaint.

The irritable nose becomes an important clinical finding in allergic disorders, particularly in children where the constant rubbing in an attempt to alleviate the itch or to reduce the sneezing produces a nasal crease (Fig.1) below the bridge of the nose which is a direct result of the ''allergic salute'' (Fig.2), the rubbing movement frequently employed to attempt to alleviate the symptoms. The observation of a nasal crease or indeed of the execution of an ''allergic salute'' is an important pointer to an underlying allergic problem and, in a Chest Clinic, can underline the diagnosis of asthma and affords a means of separating many cases of asthma from simple recurring infections.

The sneezy dripping nose always raises the question of infection and frequently a tag of ''recurring cold'' is attached to a child with

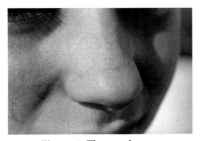

Figure 1: The nasal crease

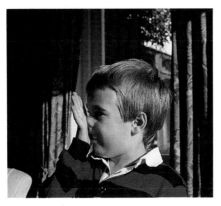

Figure 2: The ''allergic salute''

this problem so that, in management terms, infection assumes prominence in the clinician's mind and an allergic base for the problem tends to recede. The importance of examining the nose cannot therefore be stressed more firmly and the link between rhinitis and allergic chest symptoms is thereby strengthened.

A blocked nose is the major complaint in those who suffer from perennial rhinitis and the mere fact that this persists for most of the year means that the symptoms are frequently accepted by the individual and therefore largely ignored. Its association with hypersensitivity to the house dust mite in a significant proportion of these individuals, particularly the young, tends not to be appreciated as readily as the cause of the blocked nose in seasonal allergic rhinitis.

Here the allergic cause is usually correctly identified but, since the pollen season is short, it is known that the symptoms will settle spontaneously as the pollen count declines and the whole problem is self limiting. The diagnosis of perennial rhinitis and its likely allergic basis emerges readily following examination of the nasal passages where swollen, wet, blue coloured, oedematous inferior turbinates, typical of rhinitis are found and other pathologies such as nasal polyps or the purulent nasal discharge associated with infection can be excluded. Hypersensitivity to the house dust mite is the commonest respiratory allergen and accounts for some 70% or more of cases of bronchial asthma so that when one reviews a population of asthmatics where house dust mite hypersensitivity is implicated, the bronchial symptoms are frequently accompanied by nasal blockage related to the associated rhinitis. It is important, therefore, to consider appropriate treatment to suppress the rhinitis once the asthmatic symptoms have been adequately controlled.

It is not uncommon for patients to remark that following the use of systemic steroids for control of acute exacerbations of their asthma, their nasal obstruction disappears and their sense of taste and smell returns, unfortunately often only temporarily. This observation can make a patient more aware that positive treatment is possible for longstanding symptoms of rhinitis so that the general quality of life can be improved further once the asthmatic symptoms have settled.

Recurring upper respiratory infections pose a major problem in pre and early school age children. Recurring infective tonsillitis with involvement of the nasal passages is a common cause of nasal obstruction and persistent cough. These episodes respond readily to antibiotic therapy and are associated with obvious enlargment of both tonsils and adenoids. The almost constant finding of upper airways inflammation in the small child presents one of the major difficulties in the diagnosis of allergic asthma since the infective elements tend to obscure the emergence of the allergic responses and, thereby, delay the diagnosis of asthma which would be expected to develop anyway in over 10% of this population.

Night-time cough is a classical presenting sign in children with bronchial hyperreactivity associated with developing allergic bronchial asthma. Obstruction of the nasal passages, however, either anteriorly by enlarged turbinates or posteriorly by enlarged adenoids, will produce mouth breathing and associated drying of the air passages. In addition, nasal obstruction frequently accompanied by a post nasal drip which can either be serous, in association with an allergic rhinitis, or purulent, in association with infection, adenoid enlargement and tonsillitis. Whatever the cause however, night-time cough will also occur. In the evaluation of this important problem in clinical practice, it is clearly relevant to assess the significance of post nasal drip in association with nasal obstruction before bronchial hyper-reactivity and asthma emerge as the likely cause. Examination of the nose which reveals anterior obstruction with enlarged oedematous turbinates will readily confirm an allergic basis for the symptoms whereas evidence of obstruction posteriorly in association with adenoid enlargement or with inflammation of the the throat directs the attention to infection. Symptoms related to bronchial hyperreactivity will respond readily to anti-allergic measures such as inhalation of sodium cromoglycate, topical inhaled steroids or the use of beta agonist preparations. If the problem is associated with rhinitis, however, a topical steroid spray to the nasal mucosa may be required with or without the use of anti-histamine particularly if the nose shows evidence of irritation, a florid rhinitis and a nasal crease.

The use of anti-histamine containing cough sedative preparations in children will exert part of their effect by reducing the allergic reaction in the nasal mucosa so that these, in association with anti-allergic drugs used to control the bronchial irritation, can enhance the management of allergic phenonoma in the upper airways.

The presence of infection in the upper airways can become critical in the differential diagnosis of allergy in the child and presumably this is associated with similar respiratory symptoms of cough, ''chestiness'' and recurring colds which are slow to clear. Where the element of infection becomes dominant with major enlargement of tonsils and adenoids and with the persistence of chronically inflamed tissue in the posterior pharynx, there is a clear case for removing the blockage in the young asthmatic by adenoidectomy and tonsillectomy. Thus, the level of chronic and persisting infection in the upper airways can be significantly reduced. Efforts can then be concentrated on the manipulation of anti-allergic therapy to effect improved control of the allergic symptoms once infection and obstruction have been largely eliminated. A child with poorly controlled asthma who suffers from recurring posterior pharyngeal infection with gross enlargement of the adenoids and the tonsils can be improved significantly and the asthma controlled more effectively following surgical intervention.

Allergic features in the nose are found to be frequent accompaniments of symptoms of allergic bronchial asthma particularly in the child. The commonest cause is hypersensitivity to the house dust mite which is probably the major influence in some 70% of domestic cases of asthma and the link with the nasal symptoms may not be readily appreciated. Nasal symptoms and the appearance of the mucosa can help to highlight the allergic basis for respiratory symptoms, particularly in the young, and chronic nasal blockage, as a result of perennial allergic rhinitis, is a common complaint amongst those with chronic asthma and deserves positive therapeutic attention.